50% OFF Ambulatory Care Nurse Test Prep Course!

Dear Customer,

Thank you for your purchase of this Ambulatory Care Nurse Study Guide. Included with your purchase is **discounted access to our online Ambulatory Care Nurse Prep Course.** Many ANCC Ambulatory Care Nurse Test courses are needlessly expensive and don't deliver enough value. Our course provides the best ACN prep material, and with discounted access, you only pay half price.

We have structured our online course to perfectly complement your printed study guide. The ACN Test Prep Course contains **in-depth lessons** that cover all the most important topics, **600 practice questions** to ensure you feel prepared, more than **300 flashcards** for studying on the go, and **100+ instructional videos**.

Online Ambulatory Care Nurse Prep Course

Topics Covered:

- Assess and Evaluate
  - Cardiovascular Assessment
  - Immunology and Oncology
  - Ear, Nose, and Throat Pathophysiology
- Plan and Communicate
  - Care Coordination
  - Respiratory Procedures and Interventions
  - Infection Control
- Professional Role
  - Patient Rights
  - Fiscal Health
  - Quality Improvement and Risk Assessment
- Education
  - Principles of Education
  - Communication
  - Cultural Competence and Characteristics

Course Features:

- Ambulatory Care Nurse Study Guide
  - Get access to content from the best reviewed study guide available.
- Track Your Progress
  - Our customized course allows you to check off content you have studied or feel confident with.
- 3 Full-Length Practice Tests
  - With 600+ practice questions and lesson reviews, you can test yourself again and again to build confidence.
- Ambulatory Care Nurse Flashcards
  - Our course includes a flashcard mode consisting of over 300 content cards to help you study.

To lock in your discounted access, visit mometrix.com/university/acn/ or simply scan this QR code with your smartphone. At the checkout page, enter the discount code: **ACN50OFF**.

If you have any questions or concerns, please contact us at support@mometrix.com.

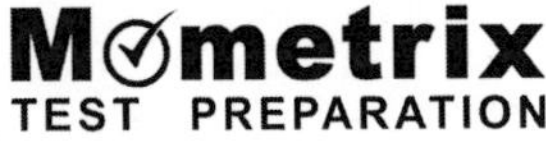

Ambulatory Care Nursing Exam Practice Questions

Ambulatory Care Nurse Practice Tests & Review for the Ambulatory Care Nursing Exam

Written and edited by the Mometrix Test Prep

Printed in the United States of America

This paper meets the requirements of ANSI/NISO Z39.48-1992 (Permanence of Paper).

Mometrix offers volume discount pricing to institutions. For more information or a price quote, please contact our sales department at sales@mometrix.com or 888-248-1219.

Paperback
ISBN 13: 978-1-5167-0581-8
ISBN 10: 1-5167-0581-5

Ebook
ISBN 13: 978-1-5167-1522-0
ISBN 10: 1-5167-1522-5

DEAR FUTURE EXAM SUCCESS STORY

First of all, **THANK YOU** for purchasing Mometrix study materials!

Second, congratulations! You are one of the few determined test-takers who are committed to doing whatever it takes to excel on your exam. **You have come to the right place.** We developed these practice tests with one goal in mind: to deliver you the best possible approximation of the questions you will see on test day.

Standardized testing is one of the biggest obstacles on your road to success, which only increases the importance of doing well in the high-pressure, high-stakes environment of test day. Your results on this test could have a significant impact on your future, and these practice tests will give you the repetitions you need to build your familiarity and confidence with the test content and format to help you achieve your full potential on test day.

Your success is our success

We would love to hear from you! If you would like to share the story of your exam success or if you have any questions or comments in regard to our products, please contact us at **800-673-8175** or **support@mometrix.com**.

Thanks again for your business and we wish you continued success!

Sincerely,
The Mometrix Test Preparation Team

Written and edited by the Mometrix Exam Secrets Test Prep Team
Printed in the United States of America

Table of Contents

Practice Test #1

1. If a patient has experienced a corneal abrasion and has much tearing, pain, and photophobia, the first intervention that the ambulatory care nurse anticipates is:

a. Eye flush with normal saline
b. Cycloplegic agent
c. Antibiotic ophthalmic ointment
d. Nonpressure eye patch

2. The plaque formation that is found with coronary artery disease results from accumulation of:

a. LDL particles
b. HDL particles
c. Triglycerides
d. Amino acids

3. If a patient is scheduled for a right breast biopsy, but no site markings are visible when the patient is draped, the ambulatory care nurse should:

a. Assume the surgeon knows the correct side.
b. Stop the procedure until the correct side is confirmed.
c. Make a note to remind staff to mark surgical sites.
d. Ask the surgeon if the side is correct.

4. When reviewing data as part of process improvement, the ambulatory care nurse notes an improvement in patient satisfaction from 78% to 92% after the addition of one new staff person. This change in satisfaction rates is probably a:

a. Random event
b. Common cause variation
c. Special-cause variation
d. Statistical aberration

5. Both before and after a splinting procedure for an extremity, the ambulatory care nurse should conduct the CSM check, which includes checking for:

a. Circulation, sensation, and movement
b. Condition, safety, and management
c. Cause, stability, and malfunctioning
d. Change, sensitivity, and maintenance

6. A truth-in-lending statement must be provided to a patient/guardian:

a. At the time a credit agreement is made
b. At the initial visit to a healthcare provider
c. If a patient indicates an inability to pay
d. If a claim has been denied by an insurance company

7. The ambulatory care nurse is concerned that staff members are not listening carefully or patiently to older patients. Which of the following interactions indicates a listening fault?

a. Staff person finishes a patient's sentences
b. Staff person asks additional questions when the patient stops speaking
c. Staff person focuses completely on the patient when the patient speaks
d. Staff person addresses questions to the patient instead of the caregiver

8. If blood specimens are drawn in the ambulatory care center and transported to a laboratory for testing, which of the following specimens must be protected from exposure to light?

a. CBC
b. Bilirubin
c. Glucose
d. Parathyroid hormone

9. When conducting a fingerstick for point of care blood glucose testing, the best finger to use is the:

a. Thumb
b. Index finger
c. 3rd or 4th finger
d. 5th (little) finger

10. A nonverbal young adult patient with autism spectrum disorder is scheduled for a minor surgical procedure and is accompanied by a parent, but the patient is very frightened, distressed, and uncooperative. The best way to reduce the patient's anxiety is to:

a. Leave the patient alone for a period of time.
b. Pat the patient on the arm and speak soothingly.
c. Ask the parent for advice about appropriate interventions.
d. Ask the parent to leave the room.

11. The primary purpose of an ambulatory care center participating in an ambulatory care registry, such as the PINNACLE Registry or the Diabetes Collaborative Registry, is to:

a. Network with other ambulatory care centers.
b. Increase rates of reimbursement.
c. Improve the quality of care.
d. Implement improved resource allocation.

12. When applying the Rule of 9s to determine the percentage of body surface area that has been burned, if an adult patient has burns covering the front of the right arm and anterior trunk (chest and abdomen), the percentage of BSA that is burned is:

a. 9%
b. 18%
c. 22.5%
d. 27%

13. The coding system that is used to code for outpatient diagnoses is:

a. ICD-9
b. HCPCS/CPT
c. ICD-10-CM
d. ICD-10-PCS

14. If an outpatient facility plans to establish a telehealth program to provide medical consultation and services to a tri-state area, the first consideration is:

a. Costs of implementation
b. State laws and regulations
c. Staffing requirements
d. Issues of reimbursement

15. In a physician's office, the encounter form typically contains:

a. A review of patient systems and health history
b. CPT and ICD-10-CM codes applicable to the type of practice
c. CPT and ICD-10-PCS codes applicable to the type of practice
d. A history of patient visits to the practice

16. A 62-year-old female patient has been having episodes of pain in the right upper quadrant of her abdomen radiating to the right scapula and persisting for periods of about 30-90 minutes. What imaging does the ambulatory care nurse anticipate?

a. Magnetic resonance imaging
b. Computed tomography
c. Radiograph
d. Ultrasound

17. A patient brings materials printed from the internet regarding a new treatment and asks the ambulatory care nurse to evaluate the information. The nurse should begin by:

a. Telling the patient to trust nothing found on the internet
b. Advising the patient to discuss the matter with the physician
c. Searching the internet for the source of the material
d. Suggesting that the patient ask a pharmacist

18. If a patient is a smoker and is to be scheduled for surgery, the patient should be advised to:

a. Decrease smoking.
b. Use a bronchodilator before surgery.
c. Stop smoking at least 6 weeks before surgery.
d. Quit smoking 24 hours before surgery.

19. The leadership style that is most likely to promote an atmosphere encouraging creativity is:

a. Authoritarian
b. Democratic
c. Bureaucratic
d. Laissez-faire

20. A clinic that serves a broad population, including a homeless population, plans to increase screening for sexually transmitted diseases in order to start earlier treatment. The most efficient method is likely to:

a. Offer screening to a target age population.
b. Take a survey to determine the target population.
c. Offer screening to high-risk individuals.
d. Offer screening to all patients.

21. If a new graduate nurse who has been practicing for fewer than 12 months seems unsure about delegated tasks and lacks good problem-solving skills, the stage of role transition that this behavior exemplifies is:

a. Knowing
b. Learning
c. Being
d. Doing

22. If a physician asks the ambulatory care nurse to make arrangements for a Medicare patient to be scheduled for a cerebral MRI, and the patient's diagnosis is diabetes mellitus, type 2, what further information is most important for the nurse prior to ordering the test?

a. Diagnosis for which the MRI is needed
b. Timeframe for ordering the MRI
c. Patient's health insurance carrier
d. Patient's concerns regarding claustrophobia

23. With goal-focused learning, the learners are presented with:

a. A goal to attain
b. A problem to solve
c. Possible outcomes
d. A case study

24. The most effective method to ensure staff members in an ambulatory care facility are prepared to carry out the disaster plan in case of emergency is to:

a. Post guidelines in prominent spots.
b. Make the complete disaster plan readily available.
c. Schedule practice/simulation drills.
d. Remind staff to review disaster plans.

25. The primary purpose of the National Performance Goals is to:

a. Promote preventive health measures.
b. Promote safe and effective care by tracking progress and improving outcomes.
c. Promote excellence in inpatient care settings.
d. Establish evidence-based practice guidelines.

26. Risk factors commonly associated with development of diabetes mellitus, type 2, include:

a. Young age and inactivity
b. Malnutrition and anemia
c. Obesity and inactivity
d. Smoking and drinking alcohol

27. After initial accreditation by the Joint Commission, an ambulatory care center should carry out the Periodic Performance Review process how often?

a. On an ongoing basis
b. Once yearly
c. 6 months prior to the next on-site survey
d. 12 months prior to the next on-site survey

28. If a patient at an ambulatory care center complains of persistent cough and is suspected of having active tuberculosis, then, according to CDC guidelines, a report must be filed with the health department within:

a. 12 hours
b. 24 hours
c. 3 days
d. 7 days

29. Which agent should be on hand in ambulatory surgery centers in order to treat an incidence of malignant hyperthermia?

a. Naloxone
b. Flumazenil
c. Dexamethasone
d. Dantrolene

30. If a healthcare organization is enrolled in the Vaccines for Children (VFC) program, the healthcare organization cannot charge a fee when administering the vaccine to a qualified child for:

a. The vaccine only
b. Administration of the vaccine
c. The office visit to obtain the vaccine
d. Any services provided at the time of the vaccination

31. The respiratory status of geriatric patients who have undergone general anesthesia for a surgical procedure should be monitored carefully because geriatric patients are especially at risk for:

a. Pneumonia
b. Pneumothorax
c. Hemothorax
d. Atelectasis

32. The primary goal of budget management should be to:

a. Describe income and outlays.
b. Prevent capital loss.
c. Show cost-effectiveness.
d. Match benchmarks.

33. If an environmental surface is contaminated with a patient's blood, which type of sterilization/disinfection process is appropriate?

a. Sterilization (such as ethylene oxide gas)
b. High-level disinfection (such as a chemical sterilant)
c. Intermediate-level disinfection (such as a chlorine-based product with tuberculocidal activity)
d. Low-level disinfection (such as chlorine-based product without tuberculocidal activity)

34. If a patient has a foreign body in the eye, the first intervention is typically to:

a. Hold the eye open by hand or with a wire eyelid speculum.
b. Evert the eyelid to examine for further foreign bodies.
c. Apply topical anesthetic to the affected eye.
d. Apply topical anesthetic to both eyes.

35. If the ambulatory care nurse is utilizing Lean-Six Sigma for quality improvement, the focus of process improvement should be on:

a. Short-term strategic goals
b. Long-term strategic goals
c. Single project goals
d. Financial goals

36. If a patient who is addicted to narcotic drugs undergoes a surgical procedure and complains of postoperative pain, the patient should receive:

a. Non-narcotic analgesia only
b. Analgesia appropriate to the type and degree of pain
c. Minimal doses of opioid analgesia
d. Maximum doses of opioid analgesia

37. A nurse resides and is licensed in state A, which is not part of the Nurse Licensure Compact, but is hired to work across the border in state B, which does participate in the NLC. If the nurse is employed in a telehealth program serving patients in 3 other states (C, D and E), all part of the NLC, the nurse must:

a. Obtain a license only for state B.
b. Use only the license from state A.
c. Obtain a license for states B and C.
d. Obtain a license for states B, C, D, and E.

38. If the ambulatory care nurse wants to look at the continuum of patient care from admission to discharge, the best method is to utilize:

a. Root cause analysis
b. Tracer methodology
c. Events and causal factors analysis
d. Force field analysis

39. When the ambulatory care nurse is assisting a nonambulatory patient to transfer from a wheelchair into an automobile, the best assistive device is likely a:

a. Lateral transfer device
b. Slip sheet
c. Sliding board
d. Transfer/pivot disc

40. If an ambulatory care practice receives an overpayment from CMS, the practice must repay the money within:

a. 90 days
b. 60 days
c. 45 days
d. 30 days

41. When doing medication reconciliation for a geriatric patient, the ambulatory care nurse is concerned that some medications or dosages may be inappropriate for elderly patients. The most efficient method of checking these medications is probably to consult:

a. PDR
b. *Drugs.com*
c. Beers Criteria
d. Drug manufacturers

42. In response to decreased renal perfusion or decreased sodium intake, the kidneys secrete:

a. Aldosterone
b. Angiotensinogen
c. Angiotensin I
d. Renin

43. The area of the ambulatory care nurse's body that is most likely to be injured when providing nursing care without the use of proper equipment is the:

a. Back
b. Shoulders
c. Hands
d. Feet

44. If a patient is pre-diabetic, hypertensive, and overweight, the best diet to recommend is the:

a. Paleo diet
b. DASH diet
c. Weight Watcher's
d. Jenny Craig

45. When an ambulatory care healthcare provider is filing a Medicare claim for durable medical equipment, which type of code is utilized?

a. ICD-10-PCS
b. HCPCS level I, CPT
c. HCPCS level II, E code
d. HCPCS level II, D code

46. One result of poor health literacy is:

a. Lower rates of hospitalization
b. Less frequent use of preventive healthcare services
c. Lower costs of health care
d. Increased use of complementary therapies

47. The type of oral diabetes medication that increases insulin secretion and may result in hypoglycemia is:

a. Biguanides
b. Thiazolidinediones
c. Alpha-glucosidase inhibitors
d. Sulfonylureas

48. The ambulatory care nurse is participating in a county-wide effort to educate parents about the importance of vaccinations for infants and children. Routine vaccinations are examples of what type of prevention?

a. Primary
b. Secondary
c. Tertiary
d. Quaternary

49. If a patient with diabetes mellitus, type 1, has been taking insulin injections four times daily and wants to decrease the frequency to twice daily, the best choice of insulin is probably:

a. Short-acting
b. Intermediate acting
c. Long-acting
d. Pre-mixed

50. Colorectal cancer screening is usually recommended for patients who are:

a. 20-50 years of age
b. 35-70 years of age
c. 50-75 years of age
d. 40-90 years of age

51. Which of the following is a risk factor for developing coronary artery or coronary heart disease?

a. Female gender
b. Tobacco exposure
c. 4-5 alcoholic drinks per week
d. Kidney disease

52. When providing instructions to a patient over the telephone, it's important for the ambulatory care nurse to:

a. Use plain language and give concise instructions.
b. Explain every step in detail, including rationale.
c. Explain all medical terms during the instructions.
d. Stop frequently during instructions to allow questions.

53. The primary problem that is associated with heart failure is dysfunction of the:

a. Right atrium
b. Right ventricle
c. Left atrium
d. Left ventricle

54. Which of the following infectious agents is NOT spread through airborne transmission?

a. Rhinovirus
b. Rubella virus
c. Influenza
d. Zika virus

55. A patient who is scheduled for angiograms with contrast should be advised that after administration of the contrast, the patient may feel:

a. Warm and as though passing urine
b. Cold and as though passing gas
c. Chills and abdominal cramping
d. Warm and chest discomfort

56. The ambulatory care nurse is creating educational materials to be displayed electronically over the internet and is concerned about linking to copyrighted material. In order to be considered copyrighted, material must:

a. Carry a copyright symbol or phrase
b. Be submitted to the government for copyright
c. Carry a statement that the material is not available for fair use
d. Be original, in a tangible medium, and creative

57. A patient who has undergone a colonoscopy should be advised to call the physician if the patient experiences:

a. Persistent abdominal pain
b. Any rectal bleeding
c. Fever over 99 °F/37.2 °C
d. Loose stool

58. The purpose of completing a hazard vulnerability assessment is to:

a. Prepare to write an all-hazards emergency plan.
b. Determine the costs involved in upgrading the all-hazards emergency plan.
c. Assign a rating score to the current all-hazards emergency plan.
d. Identify gaps in the current all-hazards emergency plan.

59. When the Rinne test for hearing deficits is conducted, sound is normally heard:

a. Twice as long through the air as through the bone
b. Twice as long through the bone as through the air
c. The same duration of time through the air as through the bone
d. Through the bone but not through the air

60. The best source of information about consumer product recalls, such as for cars seats, is:

a. Centers for Disease Control and Prevention
b. Consumer Product Safety Commission
c. Agency for Toxic Substances and Disease Registry
d. Environmental Protection Agency

61. According to Occupational Safety and Health Administration (OSHA) regulations, if a workplace-related injury results in hospitalization, loss of an eye, or amputation, OSHA must be notified within:

a. 72 hours
b. 48 hours
c. 24 hours
d. 12 hours

62. A patient who was having lab work prior to chemotherapy became very angry when the needle puncture hurt and insisted to the ambulatory care nurse that the lab technician was incompetent, to which the nurse replied, "It sounds as though that triggered a lot of feelings." This is an example of:

a. De-escalating
b. Redirecting
c. Side-tracking
d. Placating

63. A patient with obstructive sleep apnea complains of difficulty falling asleep with the CPAP device because the pressure feels uncomfortable. The best suggestion is likely for the patient to:

a. Wait until very sleepy to apply the mask.
b. Use the ramp function.
c. Decrease the pressure.
d. Try a different type of mask.

64. If a young adult patient states, "I just can't let my parents know that I am pregnant. They will be so upset," which of the following is a therapeutic response that shows active empathetic listening?

a. "You feel afraid that your parents won't be supportive."
b. "You believe you can't tell your parents."
c. "What is the worst that could happen if you tell them?"
d. "I'm sure that your parents will get over it."

65. If an older adult with Alzheimer's begins to exhibit repetitive verbal and physical behavior, such as repeatedly yelling, "Help, help, help, help" and trying to leave, the best way for the ambulatory care nurse to deal with this behavior is usually with:

a. Physical restraints
b. Chemical restraints
c. Diversion
d. Reasoning

66. If a patient has a diagnosis of macular degeneration with vision impairment and the ambulatory care nurse must provide information about treatment, the nurse should:

a. Provide all information verbally.
b. Ask the patient about the degree of vision impairment.
c. Provide information in large print.
d. Provide both verbal and print information.

67. An older patient complains of chronic constipation, which the patient has been self-managing with stimulant laxatives and enemas. The patient has been advised to stop using these treatments. The best initial approach to resolve chronic constipation is:

a. Increased dietary fiber
b. Bulk laxatives
c. Magnesium-containing laxatives
d. Surfactant laxatives (stool softeners)

68. If an ambulatory care nurse in a correctional facility is interviewing a prisoner who has been diagnosed with antisocial personality disorder and the patient states that the other healthcare providers have repeatedly failed to treat his health problems, the nurse should:

a. File a complaint.
b. Tell the patient he is lying.
c. Attempt to verify the patient's complaints.
d. Ignore the patient.

69. A group in which all members share certain traits, such as all patients with heart disease, is classified as a(n):

a. Heterogeneous group
b. Homogeneous group
c. Task group
d. Closed group

70. A primary obstacle to implementing shared governance at all levels within the nursing department of an ambulatory care center is:

a. Differing levels of knowledge/experience
b. Reluctance to participate
c. Time required for participation
d. Distrust of administrative motives

71. If a patient is receiving moderate sedation for an invasive procedure, the patient should:

a. Respond to verbal commands although sometimes slowly.
b. Arouse after repeated or painful stimuli.
c. Not respond to stimuli.
d. Respond normally.

72. According to the Needlestick Safety and Prevention Act (2000), each institution must maintain a needlestick and injury log that includes (1) a description of how the incident occurred and the extent of the injury, (2) the brand and type of product involved, and (3):

a. Insurance information of the injured party
b. Referral to the state workers' compensation board
c. Assignment of blame for the incident
d. The location where the incident occurred

73. In the initial or orientation phase of a group for which the ambulatory care nurse is serving in the role of leader, the nurse is expected to:

a. Act as facilitator
b. Resolve conflicts
c. Foster cohesiveness
d. Promote trust

74. If a patient at an urgent care center suffers peritonitis because the triage ambulatory care nurse fails to recognize symptoms of acute appendicitis and requires the patient to wait for three hours before seeing a physician, the type of negligence the nurse is exhibiting is:

a. Gross negligence
b. Negligent conduct
c. Contributory negligence
d. Comparative negligence

75. If an ambulatory care nurse has received a verbal order for a medication, but the physician is called away and not available to authenticate the order, Medicare regulations allow which of the following to do so?

a. Nurse practitioner
b. Physician's assistant
c. Nurse receiving the order
d. Covering physician

76. If an older patient complains of urinary frequency and urgency, increasing shortness of breath, pain in the right knee when walking prolonged distances, and chronic constipation, the order of priority (most critical to least) should be:

a. Urinary frequency and urgency, shortness of breath, pain in right knee, chronic constipation
b. Chronic constipation, shortness of breath, urinary frequency and urgency, and pain in the right knee
c. Shortness of breath, urinary frequency and urgency, chronic constipation, and pain in the right knee
d. Pain in right knee, shortness of breath, urinary frequency and urgency, and chronic constipation

77. If the ambulatory care nurse believes that the staff of a busy clinic could reduce stress by managing time better, the first place to begin is by:

a. Asking staff to complete time logs
b. Asking for input from others
c. Advising staff they could use time more effectively
d. Setting an example

78. If intergroup conflict between two different groups of staff members is causing low morale and increased turnover in the workplace and the ambulatory care nurse wants to help to resolve the conflict, the first step in de-escalation is to:

a. Arrange for outside help.
b. Identify the conflict boundaries.
c. Consider alternate strategies.
d. Suggest a compromise.

79. If an ambulatory care nurse wants to practice a complementary therapy with patients, the first thing that the nurse should do is to:

a. Review the state nurse practice act.
b. Obtain certification for the therapies.
c. Develop an informed consent form.
d. Study the therapies.

80. If a patient tells the ambulatory care nurse in a physician's office that they are moving to another state and wants medical records to be sent to a physician who will be assuming care of the patient, the nurse should:

a. Advise the patient to tell the physician to request the records.
b. Ask the patient to sign an authorization to release medical records.
c. Provide copies of all records directly to the patient to take to the physician.
d. Assure the patient that the records will be sent to the new physician.

81. The primary problem when screening patients via telephone is:

a. Patient's lack of medical terminology
b. Deciding on the right questions
c. Time required
d. Lack of adequate nonverbal feedback

82. If an ambulatory care center is located near a major highway junction and traffic, braking, and honking sounds are evident in the waiting and examination areas, the best solution may be to:

a. Warn patients about the noise.
b. Provide background music or white noise.
c. Avoid scheduling patients during rush hour.
d. Expect patients will get used to the noise.

83. Which of the following acts establishes standards for minimum wage and overtime pay?

a. Fair Labor Standards Act
b. Contract Work Hours and Safety Standards Act
c. McNamara-O'Hara Service Contract Act
d. Civil Rights Act (1964)

84. If an ambulatory care nurse writes negative comments about their place of employment on a personal social media site that allows public access, such as Facebook, the ambulatory care nurse is likely to:

a. Do so without concern because of privacy laws.
b. Gain or lose followers.
c. Be subject to disciplinary action.
d. Be arrested and fined.

85. During telephone triage, the patient complains of lower back pain (4 on a 0-10 scale) accompanied by frequent, burning urination. Which action is most appropriate?

a. Call 911 for emergency treatment
b. Stat appointment within 1 hour
c. Same-day appointment
d. Next-day appointment

86. If an elderly patient comes to an outpatient clinic because of multiple contusions and cuts, and the patient tells the ambulatory care nurse that a family member has pushed her down the stairs, but the patient doesn't want to report the family member, the ambulatory nurse:

a. Must report the abuse to the appropriate authorities
b. Must respect the patient's wishes
c. Should ask to the caregiver about the charges
d. Should threaten to call the police if more abuse occurs

87. Which of the following infectious diseases are classified by the CDC as "standard" and requires electronic notification within the next reporting cycle?

a. SARS-associated coronavirus
b. Measles
c. Rubella
d. Gonorrhea

88. If the ambulatory care nurse inadvertently charts a telephone order and medication administration for one patient on the wrong patient's electronic health record (although the right patient got the medication), the correct procedure is to:

a. Delete the entries.
b. Leave the entries and indicate they are errors.
c. Leave the entries and write explanation in free text.
d. Delete the entries with explanation in free text.

89. When educating a patient with mild cognitive impairment (MCI) about wound care, one way to deal with the communication barrier is to:

a. Also instruct a caregiver.
b. Write everything down.
c. Break instructions into small steps.
d. Repeat the instructions numerous times.

90. If a woman in active labor comes to the emergency department without insurance or means to pay for care, the emergency department staff:

a. May screen and transfer the patient to another facility
b. May immediately transfer the woman to another facility
c. May refuse to admit the woman as a patient
d. Must deliver the child and placenta before transfer

91. If a patient in a clinic has a severe anaphylactic reaction to the Tdap immunization, the event must be reported to:

a. National Vaccine Injury Compensation Program
b. National Vaccine Program Office (NVPO)
c. Local public health department
d. Vaccine Adverse Event Reporting System (VAERS)

92. If a patient scheduled for a liver biopsy at an ambulatory surgery center lists the religion as Jehovah's Witness, the ambulatory care nurse should ask the patient about:

a. Receiving blood products
b. Dietary restrictions
c. Desire for presence of healers
d. Medication restrictions

93. If a patient has a foreign body in the eye, and it is visible and does not appear to be imbedded, the best method to remove the foreign body is by:

a. Irrigating the eye with NS until the foreign body washes out
b. Rolling moistened cotton-tipped applicator over foreign body to remove
c. Dabbing at the foreign body with a moistened gauze square
d. Using a 27-gauge needle (bevel side up) to dislodge the foreign body

94. While shared governance focuses primarily on empowering nursing, partnership councils focus on:

a. Physicians
b. Non-medical personnel
c. Members at all levels
d. Department heads

95. Before a surgical procedure can be carried out, the ambulatory care nurse should check the patient's health record to ensure that which of the following documents are in the record?

a. History, physical exam, and signed consent form
b. Problem list and signed consent form
c. Laboratory results, history, and signed consent form
d. Physical exam, problem list, and signed consent form

96. The purpose of MedWatch is to:

a. Facilitate voluntary reporting of adverse events associated with a medical products.
b. Provide lists of physicians and institutions with malpractice claims.
c. Send out alerts to physicians for drug recalls.
d. Alert healthcare providers to new drugs on the market.

97. If a patient requests copies of personal health information contained in an electronic health record at a physician's office, the office should provide the copies the patient has requested within:

a. 24 hours
b. One week
c. 30 days
d. 60 days

98. If a patient wants to complete an advance directive and asks for information, the patient should be advised to:

a. Write out the information longhand or by type.
b. Obtain a form that complies with federal guidelines.
c. Obtain any generic advance directive form.
d. Obtain a form that complies with state guidelines.

99. When carrying out rapid assessment of a patient as part of triage, the first thing to evaluate is:

a. Mental status
b. Perfusion
c. Pulse
d. Respirations

100. If a number of patients arrive simultaneously at an urgent care center—(1) man with fractured femur, (2) pregnant woman with severe vaginal bleeding, (3) child with cough and slight fever, and (4) woman with a possible stroke—the order in which the patients should be seen is:

a. 2, 4, 1, and 3
b. 2, 3, 4, and 1
c. 4, 2, 1, and 3
d. 3, 2, 4, and 1

101. A 72-year-old patient complains of increasing fatigue, weakness, and dyspnea on exertion and lack of interest in activities. The patient's pulse rate shows an increase from 70 to 96, blood pressure from 126/78 to 150/96 and respirations from 18 to 26 three minutes after activity, a likely nursing diagnosis is:

a. Risk prone health behaviors
b. Ineffective coping
c. Activity intolerance
d. Anxiety

102. When examining and cleansing a wound on a toddler's hand, the best position for the child is:

a. In the caregiver's arms in a hug hold
b. Lying supine on an examination table
c. Standing on the examination table
d. Restrained on a nurse assistant's lap

103. The medication reconciliation process should be carried out with a patient in a physician's office:

a. On admission only
b. At least annually
c. Every 4-5 visits
d. Every visit

104. If a patient presents with complaints of an allergic reaction to a bee sting, the first question that the triage nurse should ask is:

a. "Do you have any shortness of breath or swelling of the tongue or throat?"
b. "How long ago did the sting occur?"
c. "Do you have hives or itching?"
d. "Have you developed nausea, vomiting, or diarrhea?"

105. For which of the following disruptive patients might a behavior contract be an appropriate tool?

a. A patient who strikes a nurse and threatens to harm the nurse's children
b. A patient who is intellectually impaired and requires almost constant care
c. A patient with Alzheimer's disease who screams at the staff members
d. A patient who repeatedly uses foul language when addressing staff members

106. For a patient who takes multiple medications, which of the following foods is most likely one that should be avoided?

a. Milk products
b. Grapefruit
c. Soy products
d. Coffee

107. For most medications, the primary difference between the brand name drug and the generic version of the drug is the:

a. Price
b. Effectiveness
c. Mode of action
d. Method of elimination

108. Sub-acute low back pain is characterized by symptoms that persist:

a. Less than 6 weeks
b. Between 6 weeks and 3 months
c. Between 3 months 6 months
d. More than 6 months

109. If a non-pregnant patient has had persistent proteinuria ranging from 90 mg/day to 300 mg/day for 3 months, the patient is at risk for the development of:

a. Hypertension and renal insufficiency
b. Cardiovascular disease
c. Bladder and kidney infections
d. Hydronephrosis

110. Which of the following vaccines is made from attenuated live viruses?

a. MMR
b. Tetanus
c. Diphtheria
d. Hib

111. If a patient complains of frequent anxiety and wants to try complementary therapy rather than medications, which of the following is most likely to provide relief?

a. Homeopathic preparations
b. Music therapy
c. Acupuncture
d. Visualization and relaxation exercises

112. The Advance Beneficiary Notice of Noncoverage (ABN) (CMS-R-131) is provided to patients to inform them that:

a. They have not yet met their annual deductible
b. Medicare will not cover an item or service
c. The physician does not accept Medicare assignment
d. The physician does not accept Medicare patients

113. If a 74-year-old patient comes to the ambulatory care center with her daughter, and the daughter begins to describe the patient's problems while the patient remains silent, the best response is to:

a. Direct questions to the daughter.
b. Ask the daughter to leave the room.
c. Direct questions directly to the patient.
d. Ask the daughter why she is speaking for the patient.

114. Patients who are taking phenytoin for seizure disorders should be advised to have regular dental care because of increased risk of:

a. Caries
b. Gingival hyperplasia
c. Tooth staining
d. Abscesses

115. If a patient complains of urinary frequency and urgency, a positive leukocyte esterase dipstick test indicates:

a. Pyuria
b. Absence of infection
c. Glycosuria
d. Proteinuria

116. If the ambulatory care nurse is teaching a patient to self-administer insulin, and the nurse has instructed the parent to divide each site (abdomen, thigh, arm) into quadrants, the patient should then be advised to use the same quadrant for:

a. One day
b. Three days
c. Four days
d. Seven days

117. A 40-year-old patient comes to the ambulatory care center after experiencing a fall and has a small cut on the forehead. Which of the following signs or symptoms may indicate a change in mental status?

a. The patient complains of slight headache
b. The patient repeatedly asks the same question
c. The patient insists that no treatment is necessary
d. The patient appears upset about the accident

118. When discussing home care for a child with the flu and a fever, the ambulatory care nurse should stress that the parent should avoid giving the child:

a. Solid foods
b. Aspirin
c. Acetaminophen
d. Hot drinks

119. When the ambulatory care nurse is screening telephone calls, a patient calls to complain of low back pain. Which of the following additional symptoms represents an emergent situation and should result in the nurse advising the patient to hang up and call 9-1-1?

a. Pain radiating down left leg
b. Fever of 38 °C (100.4 °F)
c. Sudden loss of bowel and bladder control
d. Burning on urination and frequency

120. If a patient was scheduled for a colonoscopy but misunderstood the directions and did not adequately complete the bowel prep and became very upset when informed the procedure would have to be delayed, the most appropriate nursing diagnosis is:

a. Fear/anxiety
b. Hopelessness
c. Ineffective self-health management
d. Deficient knowledge

121. When collecting a throat specimen for the rapid strep test, the correct procedure is to:

a. Ask the patient to swab the back of the throat.
b. Ask the patient to rinse the mouth with water before collecting a specimen.
c. Swab the back of the throat, including reddened areas or pustules.
d. Swab the back of the throat, avoiding areas of pustules.

122. If the ambulatory care nurse is to administer eye drops to a patient, but drainage and crusts are evident along the eyelid margins and inner canthus, the first step is to:

a. Ask the patient to scrub the eyes.
b. Scrub the eyes by wiping back and forth with a warm damp cloth.
c. Irrigate the eyes with warm water.
d. Soak the crusts with a warm damp cloth or cotton ball, then wipe clean.

123. Following a surgical procedure at an ambulatory surgery center, the patient must be taught to use a flow-oriented incentive spirometer. Which of the following can be delegated to unlicensed assistive personnel (UAP)?

a. Assessing patient's use of spirometer
b. Monitoring the patient's frequency of using the spirometer
c. Teaching skill of using the spirometer
d. Evaluating the patient's response to the use of the spirometer

124. When fitting a patient for crutches, measure from 2 inches below the axilla to:

a. The top of the foot
b. 2 inches in front of the patient
c. 6 inches in front of the patient
d. 6 inches to the side of the patient

125. An older patient tells the ambulatory care nurse that she has no telephone service because of limited income. The nurse is aware that the Lifeline service is available to low-income individuals who meet specific criteria, which can include:

a. Medicare recipient
b. Income below 150% of poverty level
c. Medicaid recipient
d. Age over 65

126. As a case manager for a stroke patient who has been discharged home but is having difficulty preparing foods because of residual right-sided weakness, the most appropriate referral is to a(n):

a. Occupational therapist
b. Physical therapist
c. Home health aide
d. Meals-on-wheels program

127. Which members of a staff in a healthcare facility must receive education regarding compliance issues?

a. Physicians and nurses
b. Administrative staff
c. Compliance officer(s)
d. All staff members

128. A patient who has received an anesthetic agent at an ambulatory surgery center must be supervised by a responsible adult following the procedure for at least:

a. 4-6 hours
b. 6-8 hours
c. 8-12 hours
d. 12-24 hours

129. The primary purpose of a "time out" prior to beginning a surgical procedure is to confirm:

a. The correct patient, procedure, and markings
b. That all necessary staff members are present
c. That all necessary equipment is available
d. The patient's name and ID number

130. The emergency power source for the ambulatory surgery center should be able to operate the lighting and equipment in operating rooms for a period of at least:

a. One hour
b. Two hours
c. Three hours
d. Four hours

131. The purpose of the Caffeine Halothane Contracture test is to determine if a patient will exhibit:

a. Caffeine allergy
b. Halothane allergy
c. Malignant hyperthermia
d. Anesthesia-associated hypotension

132. Which of the following findings indicates hypothyroidism associated with disease in the pituitary gland?

a. Decreased TSH and decreased free T4
b. Elevated TSH and decreased free T4
c. Elevated TSH and elevated free T4
d. Decreased TSH and elevated free T4

133. If the ambulatory care nurse is to collect a wound specimen for culture and sensitivities, the correct procedure is to collect the specimen from:

a. Wound drainage
b. About the wound perimeter
c. Inside the wound
d. Inside and outside the wound

134. If a patient is scheduled for an abdominal CT with IV contrast, it is important to ask the patient about allergies to:

a. Metals
b. Eggs
c. Milk products
d. Iodine

135. A patient scheduled for cardiac stress testing should be advised to avoid caffeine for:

a. 4 hours before the test
b. 8 hours before the test
c. 12 hours before the test
d. 24 hours before the test

136. According to the National Institute for Occupational Safety and Health (NIOSH) Hierarchy of Controls for exposure to workplace hazards, which of the following interventions is the most effective?

a. Elimination of the hazard
b. Engineering controls
c. Substitution
d. Administrative controls

137. The ethnic group that has the highest prevalence of asthma is:

a. Caucasian
b. African American
c. Asian
d. Polynesian

138. Females should be screened for cervical cancer every:

a. 1 year from ages 21-65
b. 2 years from ages 21-75
c. 3 years from ages 21-65
d. 4 years from ages 16-65

139. The BMI that indicates a patient is overweight is:

a. 18.5-24.9
b. 25-29.9
c. 30-39.9
d. Over 40

140. A 13-year-old boy complains of intermittent bilateral pain in the thigh and lower leg in the evening and at night, but an examination shows no abnormality. These symptoms are consistent with:

a. Deep vein thrombosis
b. Growing pains
c. Nocturnal leg cramps
d. Chronic compartment syndrome

141. If both spouses have separate family insurance policies that cover the spouse and children with coordination of benefits provisions, which spouse's insurance is primary?

a. Either spouse
b. Both spouses (both insurance policies will pay)
c. The spouse whose birthday comes first in the year
d. The spouse whose birthday comes last in the year

142. If a patient is receiving methotrexate as a chemotherapeutic agent, which antidote may be co-administered to decrease adverse effects of methotrexate?

a. Penicillamine
b. Sodium thiosulphate
c. Phentolamine
d. Leucovorin calcium

143. If a patient states she plans to take St. John's Wort for mild depression rather than an SSRI, the ambulatory care nurse should:

a. Advise the patient that SSRIs are more effective.
b. Carefully review the patient's list of medications.
c. Suggest the patient consider taking both.
d. Advise the patient that St. John's Wort is ineffective.

144. If a patient comes to the ambulatory care center complaining of chest pain and shortness of breath, the first action of the ambulatory care nurse should be to:

a. Take the patient by wheelchair to an examination room.
b. Ask the patients questions about the quality of the pain.
c. Take the patient's vital signs.
d. Administer oxygen to the patient.

145. If a patient faints while awaiting an examination at an ambulatory care center and complains of feeling very weak and faint after regaining consciousness, the ambulatory nurse should place the patient in:

a. Flat supine position
b. Semi-Fowler's position
c. Trendelenburg position
d. Upright position

146. When using the post-anesthesia recovery score (also known as the modified Aldrete score) of 0 to 10 to determine a patient's readiness for discharge, PACU discharge requires a score of:

a. 0-2
b. 3-5
c. 6-8
d. 9-10

147. A patient comes to the ambulatory care center 10 minutes after being stung by a bee. The patient is developing rapid generalized edema and shortness of breath. The treatment that the nurse anticipates is:

a. Steroid
b. Epinephrine
c. Oxygen
d. Diuretic

148. Following a minor surgical procedure for which the patient received moderate ("conscious") sedation, the patient should expect to be discharged after:

a. 30-40 minutes
b. 1-2 hours
c. 3-4 hours
d. 5-6 hours

149. Following a surgical procedure in which the patient received moderate sedation, the patient's blood pressure drops to 85/48 from a preoperative level of 126/84. The initial response is usually to:

a. Increase intravenous fluids.
b. Administer an antihypertensive drug.
c. Place the patient in Trendelenburg position.
d. Administer naloxone.

150. When assessing key performance measures as part of the ambulatory care process improvement assessment, which of the following relates to access to care?

a. FTE support staff per MD
b. Rejection/Denial rate of insurance
c. Immunization rates
d. Average telephone wait time

Answer Key and Explanations for Test #1

1. B: The first intervention that the ambulatory care nurse anticipates is a cycloplegic agent, such as cyclopentolate 1%, to relieve the pain and spasms. This is generally followed by an antibiotic ophthalmic ointment, such as erythromycin (if not related to contact lenses) or tobramycin (if related to contact lenses). Corneal abrasion results from direct scratching or scraping trauma to the eye, often involving contact lenses, causing a defect in the epithelium of the cornea. Infection with corneal ulceration can occur with abrasions.

2. A: The plaque formation that is found with coronary artery disease results from the accumulation of LDL particles in the endothelium. LDL penetrates the arteries and becomes oxidized by free radicals, leading to an inflammatory reaction in which monocytes enter the epithelium, becoming macrophages and attempting to phagocytize the LDL. The LDL that builds up in the macrophages causes them to transform into "foam cells" that remain within the endothelium and over which fibrotic tissue forms.

3. B: If a patient is scheduled for a right breast biopsy but no site markings are visible when the patient is draped, the ambulatory care nurse should stop the procedure until the correct side is confirmed. The purpose of site markings is to doublecheck that the correct side is being operated on, so the markings should be visible after draping is applied. If not, then the records must be checked to verify the correct side and the patient examined to determine if the incorrect side was marked.

4. C: If, when reviewing data as part of process improvement, the ambulatory care nurse notes an improvement in patient satisfaction from 76% to 92% after the addition of one new staff person, this change in satisfaction rates is probably a special-cause variation. While common-cause variation occurs by chance, a special-cause variation directly relates to some event or change. In this case, the increase in satisfaction rates likely results from the addition of a new staff member.

5. A: Both before and after a splinting procedure for an extremity, the ambulatory care nurse should conduct the CSM check, which includes checking for:

- **Circulation**: Checking the strength of the distal pulse, capillary refill time, and skin color.
- **Sensation**: Checking the patient's ability to feel and any pain, tingling or burning sensations.
- **Movement**: Ensuring that the patient can move the fingers or toes of the affected limb.

6. A: The credit agreement includes the total amount owed, the payment schedule, and amounts that have been agreed upon (usually monthly payments). If a patient simply notifies the healthcare provider of the intention to make payments and does so without discussing the matter with the healthcare provider, then no formal agreement is necessary. However, if the healthcare provider or staff discusses the matter with the patient/guardian and sets up a schedule of payments, a formal written agreement is required. The credit agreement may include interest charges and charges for late payments.

7. A: A listening fault occurs when the staff person does not take the time to listen properly. Listening faults include finishing a patient's sentence if they pause, have trouble finding words, or speak slowly. Another type of listening fault is to interrupt the patient in the middle of sentences to make comments or ask questions instead of waiting until the patient has finished speaking. Another listening fault is to show a lack of interest, by looking bored, looking away, or mumbling a vague response.

8. B: If blood specimens are drawn in the ambulatory care center and transported to a laboratory for testing, the specimen that must be protected from exposure to light is the bilirubin specimen, as the bilirubin level may decrease by 50% within 60 minutes of light exposure. If a special container is not available for the specimen vial, then it can be wrapped in aluminum foil for transport. Other light-sensitive specimens include vitamins B_1, B_6, B_{12} and C as well as carotene, red cell folate, and serum folate.

9. C: When conducting a fingerstick for point of care blood glucose testing, the best finger to use is the 3rd or 4th fingertip. The ambulatory care nurse should examine the fingertip and the grain of the fingerprints and should use the lancet across the grain rather than parallel to the grain, on the side of the finger pad. A drop of blood should be collected on the test strip and read by the monitor following manufacturer's directions as they may vary slightly. A normal blood glucose reading is below 100 mg/dL.

10. C: If a nonverbal young adult patient with autism spectrum disorder is scheduled for a minor surgical procedure and is accompanied by a parent, but the patient is very frightened, distressed, and uncooperative, the best way to reduce the patient's anxiety is to ask the parent for advice about appropriate interventions. The parent likely knows what triggers the patient's anxiety and what has a calming effect. Generally, touching a patient with autism spectrum disorder without asking first can be very distressing to the patient.

11. C: The primary purpose is to improve the quality of care for the practice and ambulatory care as a whole. Participation allows participants to benchmark their own quality level. Registries help to track and improve care for specific types of disease. Participation in some registries is mandatory, but outpatient registries usually ask for voluntary participation.

12. C: When applying the Rule of 9s to determine the percentage of body surface area that has been burned, if an adult patient has burns covering the front of the right arm (4.5%) and anterior trunk (chest and abdomen) (18%), the percentage of BSA that is burned is 22.5%. Rule of 9s:

- Head/neck: 9% (4.5% front, 4.5% back)
- Anterior trunk: 18%
- Posterior trunk: 18%
- Leg: 18% (9% front, 9% back)
- Arm: 9% (4.5% front, 4.5% back)
- Genitals: 1%

13. C: The coding system that is used to code for outpatient diagnoses is ICD-10-CM. The same coding system is used to code for inpatient diagnoses as well, so there is consistency when patients transfer from one level of care to another. ICD-10-CM replaced ICD-9 in October 2015. Inpatient and outpatient services, however, use different coding systems for procedures. Inpatient facilities utilized ICD-10-PCS, and outpatient facilities utilized HCPCS/CPT. HCPCS level I codes incorporate the CPT codes, but level II codes are used for services not included as part of the CPT codes, such as ambulance service.

14. B: If an outpatient facility plans to establish a telehealth program to provide medical consultation and services to a tri-state area, the first consideration is state laws and regulations, as these may vary considerably. Some states require informed consent while others do not, and in some cases the telepresenter must be present with the patient when obtaining the consent. Some states require an initial in-person visit before patients can receive telehealth services. License portability is often an issue because many states require those providing telehealth services to be licensed in the state where the patient is residing.

15. B: In a physician's office, the encounter form typically contains CPT (procedure) and ICD-10-CM (diagnosis) codes applicable to the type of practice. The encounter form is completed by the healthcare provider during visits. The encounter form then serves as the basis for billing. Each type of practice creates its own encounter form or uses a corresponding standardized form. Because there are very many CPT and ICD-10-CM codes, one form cannot contain them all, so a practice chooses the codes that most apply to the procedures and diagnoses of that practice.

16. D: These symptoms are consistent with cholelithiasis, and an ultrasound will show whether gallstones are present. Gallstones are more common in females than males and in those older than age 60.

17. C: If a patient brings materials printed from the internet regarding a new treatment and asks the ambulatory care nurse to evaluate the information, the nurse should begin by searching the internet for the source of the material. This presents a good opportunity to educate the patient about the importance of a valid source and how to determine validity. If the source and information is valid, the nurse should suggest the patient discuss the treatment with the physician.

18. C: If a patient is a smoker and is to be scheduled for surgery, the patient should be advised to stop smoking at least 6 weeks before surgery if possible (and 6 weeks after surgery as well). Smokers have higher risks of morbidity and mortality associated with surgery. Nicotine is a vasoconstrictor, and this can interfere with oxygenation and healing of tissues. Anesthesiologists should always be aware of a patient's smoking status prior to surgery.

19. B: The leadership style that is most likely to promote an atmosphere encouraging creativity is democratic. Because all members are encouraged to participate and to find solutions to problems, this encourages members to think creatively. While democratic leadership may delay decision-making because of the need to include the ideas of many, the solutions are often more effective because of the time taken to discuss issues and reach consensus. However, it can be challenging to get people from different backgrounds and levels of education to work together cooperatively.

20. D: If a clinic that serves a broad population plans to increase screening for sexually transmitted diseases, including HIV, in order to start earlier treatment, the most efficient method is likely to offer screenings to all patients. While patients aged 15-24 account for about 50% of those with sexually transmitted diseases, rates have been rising for those over age 50. Injection drug users, many of whom are homeless, have increased risk of not only bloodborne infections, such as HIV, but other sexually transmitted diseases as well.

21. D: The three stages of role transition that usually occur over about 12 months include:

- Doing (3-4 months): The new nurse experiences some shock at the realities of work and recognizes limitations. The nurse is often unsure about delegated tasks and lacks good problem-solving skills.
- Being (4-5 months): The nurse may feel increased stress but also more awareness of personal role and may question and search for answers although the nurse may feel unprepared for the position.
- Knowing (3-4 months): The nurse gains confidence and accepts new role.

22. A: While all of these are considerations, the most important information when ordering the test is the diagnosis for which the MRI is needed. Diagnostic procedures must be properly coded for both the procedure and the probable diagnosis. For example, an ICD-10-CM diagnostic code must be applied for every procedure, but an MRI is not a routine procedure associated with diabetes, so that diagnosis would not be acceptable.

23. A: With goal-focused learning, the learners are presented with a goal to attain so that the learners have a very clear idea of what they must accomplish. Goal-focused learning is frequently used for learning processes. For example, goal-focused learning may be used when teaching a patient to self-administer insulin. With goal-focused learning, all materials and instructions are geared toward achieving the goal that has been identified. With goal-focused learning, the learner should be advised exactly what constitutes successful attainment of the goal.

24. C: The most effective method to ensure staff members in an ambulatory care facility are prepared to carry out the disaster plan in case of emergency is to schedule practice/simulation drills. Simulations may include fire drills to determine if the staff knows how to protect patients, contain small blazes, and evacuate. More extensive simulations may include various scenarios with volunteer "patients" and simulated injuries. Prior to the simulations, the staff members should be educated about the disaster plan and should review established protocols.

25. B: The primary purpose of the National Patient Safety Goals (NPSGs) is to track progress to allow for measurable outcomes which results in safer and more efficient patient care. These goals are broken down into chapters by specialty. The Ambulatory Health Care chapter focuses specifically on patient identification, medication safety, infection prevention, health outcomes, and preventing mistakes in surgery. For all inpatient accreditation programs, the NPSGs were replaced by the National Performance Goals, so NPSGs now apply only to outpatient accreditation programs.

26. C: Risk factors commonly associated with development of diabetes mellitus, type 2, include obesity and inactivity. Risk also increases with a family history of diabetes. Risk increases with age, possibly because of the tendency to gain weight and exercise less, although dietary changes have resulted in a substantial increase in the rates of diabetes among children and adolescents. Diet may increase risk, especially a diet high in simple carbohydrates, and diabetes risk increases with high levels of triglycerides (which reflect carbohydrate intake).

27. A: After initial accreditation by the Joint Commission, an ambulatory care center should carry out the Periodic Performance Review process on an ongoing basis to ensure that the center continues to meet the standards set by the joint Commission. The Periodic Performance Review process is also completed as preparation for the initial accreditation, which occurs within one year after the application for accreditation is filed.

28. B: If a patient at an ambulatory care center complains of persistent cough and is suspected of having active tuberculosis, then, according to CDC guidelines, a report must be filed with the health department within 24 hours because of the risk of transmission. If a latent case of tuberculosis is suspected or confirmed, the health department must be notified within 3 days. State regulations may vary regarding reporting of patients who are nonadherent to treatment.

29. D: Dantrolene is the agent that should be on hand in an ambulatory surgery center in order to treat an incidence of malignant hyperthermia. Dantrolene is usually given initially at a dose of 2.5 mg/kg, with an additional 1 mg/kg repeated every five minutes until symptoms, up to the maximum total dose of 10 mg/kg. Other treatments may include cooling blankets to help lower body temperature and IV fluids to maintain renal function. Hyperkalemia is common.

30. A: If a healthcare organization is enrolled in the Vaccines for Children (VFC) program, the healthcare organization cannot charge a fee when administering the vaccine for the vaccine itself as the vaccines are provided without cost to the participating healthcare provider. However, the healthcare provider can charge a fee for administration of the vaccine and may charge for the office visit or any additional services provided. Free vaccinations are available to children younger than 19 who meet eligibility requirements.

31. D: The respiratory status of geriatric patients who have undergone general anesthesia for a surgical procedure should be monitored carefully because geriatric patients are especially at risk for atelectasis because of hypoventilation, post-anesthesia narcosis, and inactivity. Patients must be instructed in the use of the incentive spirometer and should be encouraged to ambulate early. Narcotics may interfere with the cough reflex so should be used cautiously and replaced with non-narcotic analgesia as soon as possible.

32. D: The primary goal of budget management should be to match benchmarks. Costs should be monitored to determine if they are in line with best practices. Budget management includes efforts to control expenses and developing plans to correct budget deficits or unexpected variances. When possible, achieving benchmarks should be rewarded in some way, such as through budgeted bonuses or time off. Budget management should include the use of various measures to control costs, and a balanced scorecard may be utilized to show results.

33. C: If an environmental surface is contaminated with a patient's blood, the type of sterilization/disinfection process that is appropriate is intermediate level disinfection, such as a chlorine-based product with tuberculocidal activity. This type of disinfectant is liquid and must be in contact with the contaminated surface for a period of at least one minute. Intermediate-level disinfectants destroy vegetative bacteria, mycobacteria, most fungi, and most viruses, but it does not destroy bacterial spores. The only process that kills all spores is sterilization.

34. D: If a patient has a foreign body in the eye, the first intervention is typically to apply topical anesthetic to both eyes so that blinking in the unaffected eye is suppressed. The next steps include:

- Hold the eye open by hand or with a wire eyelid speculum.
- Carefully remove the foreign body with a small-gauge needle or a moistened cotton swab.
- Note: Rust rings from metallic objects should be removed with an ophthalmic burr (if not over the pupil), and the patient is referred to an ophthalmologist for further rust ring removal within 24 hours.
- Evert the eyelid and examine the eye carefully for further foreign bodies.
- Treat abrasions as indicated.

35. B: If the ambulatory care nurse is utilizing Lean-Six Sigma for quality improvement, the focus of process improvement should be on long-term (usually at least 1-3 years) strategic goals, so the aim is to change the culture to facilitate permanent change. The four characteristics include (1) establishing strategies to achieve long-term goals, (2) creating an underlying belief in performance improvement throughout the organization, (3) reducing costs through quality, and (4) incorporating improvement methodology, such as PDSA.

36. B: If a patient who is addicted to narcotic drugs undergoes a surgical procedure and complains of postoperative pain, the patient should receive analgesia appropriate to the type and degree of pain. Even patients who are addicted to narcotics have the right to pain control although they may require larger doses than normal because of tolerance. However, some patients who were formerly addicted may refuse narcotics because of the fear that they will resume drug use.

37. D: If a nurse resides and is licensed in state A but works in state B and provides telehealth services to states C, D, and E, the nurse must obtain separate licenses for states B, C, D, and E because the Nurse Licensure Compact does not apply to the nurse since the nurse's primary residence is in a state that is not part of the compact. The NLC applies to RNs, LVNs, LPNs, and most recently (as of 2020) to APRNs. APRNs have a separate compact (the APRN compact) which currently is active across 7 states.

38. B: If the ambulatory care nurse wants to look at the continuum of patient care from admission to discharge, the best method is to utilize tracer methodology. With this method, on patient is selected and the experiences of the patient at every step in treatment and care are evaluated. For example, if a patient received occupational therapy, the nurse would ask as many clarifying questions as possible: how the order is obtained, how the appointment is set, how the patient is transported, how the service is rendered, how treatment is documented, how follow-up is planned, and how treatment is billed.

39. C: When the ambulatory care nurse is assisting a nonambulatory patient to transfer from a wheelchair into an automobile, the best assistive device is likely a sliding board. Newer sliding boards have a round disc on which the patient is seated, and this disc then slides along the board so that the friction during transfer is not on the patient's tissue. Slip sheets are used to reposition patients. The lateral transfer device aids in lateral transfers, such as from the bed to a gurney. Transfer/pivot discs are circular discs on which a patient stands and is then pivoted to sit.

40. B: If an ambulatory care practice receives an overpayment from CMS, the practice must repay the money within 60 days, according to provisions of the False Claims Act. Failure to do so may result in penalties corresponding to three times the loss and up to $11,000 per claim. The government may recover any money that was paid as the result of claims that were false or fraudulent. False claims are those that the entity knows or should know are violations, such as claims for care not rendered, care already billed for, miscoding/upcoding, and services not supported by documentation. Fraudulent claims may also result from referrals made in violation of the Physician Self-Referral Law (the Stark Law) and the Anti-Kickback Statute.

41. C: The Beers Criteria (American Geriatric Society) lists drugs that are inappropriate for older adults. The Beers Criteria can be incorporated into clinical decision support systems so that alerts are issued if a medication or dosage is inappropriate for the patient. The Beers Criteria lists the organ system/therapeutic category of the drugs, the rationale for including the drugs on the list, the recommendations (conditions for avoidance and exceptions), the quality and strength of evidence as well as references.

42. D: In response to decreased renal perfusion or decreased sodium intake, the kidneys secrete renin into the circulatory system. Renin then converts angiotensinogen (produced by the liver) into angiotensin I. A pulmonary enzyme (angiotensin-converting enzyme) then further converts the angiotensin I to angiotensin II, which stimulates the production and release of aldosterone by the adrenal glands. Aldosterone functions to conserve sodium and increase excretion of potassium in order to increase blood pressure by increasing the volume of extracellular fluid.

43. A: The area of the body that is most likely to be injured when providing nursing care without the use of proper equipment is the back. Back injuries occur from lifting and repositioning patients. Ideally, mechanical lifts and other equipment should always be available and a no-lifting policy in place in order to prevent strain on the muscles. Slip sheets should be used to reposition patients in bed, and at least two people should carry out the repositioning.

44. B: If a patient is pre-diabetic, hypertensive, and overweight, the best diet to recommend is the DASH diet as it has proven effective for these three conditions. The DASH diet includes 3 meals and 2 snacks so patients are less likely to feel hungry. The diet focuses on vegetables, lean protein-rich foods, low-fat dairy products, and nuts and seeds. The newest version of the diet is more restrictive of grains than previous versions, and patients are advised to avoid sugared products in favor of fresh fruit.

45. C: When an ambulatory care healthcare provider is filing a Medicare claim for durable medical equipment, the type of code that is utilized is HCPCS level II E code. ICD-10-PCS is used to code for procedures and equipment for patients in hospitals. Most procedures for ambulatory care are coded with HCPCS level I CPT codes, but some things use HCPCS level II codes. D codes, for example, are used for dental procedures with code sets copyrighted by the American Dental Association.

46. B: One result of poor health literacy is less frequent use of preventive healthcare services, often because people are unaware of the need for these services. Other results include higher rates of hospitalization and higher costs for healthcare, partially because treatment is delayed, resulting in more complications, or preventive services is not utilized. Patients with poor health literacy often have very poor understanding of chronic conditions and the care necessary and may feel ashamed.

47. D: Sulfonylureas are the type of diabetes medication that increases insulin secretion by stimulating beta cells in the pancreas and may result in hypoglycemia, especially if the patient's dietary intake is insufficient or the dosage is too high. Sulfonylureas include tolbutamide, glipizide, and glimepiride, with some short-acting and some long-acting. Sulfonylureas should not be used if there is no residual production of insulin. Sulfonylureas may be used a monotherapy but are often combined with other drugs, such as metformin (in the class biguanides).

48. A: Routine vaccinations are an example of primary prevention because the goal is to prevent disease or injury through preventive action. Primary preventive efforts are usually aimed at the general population or large subsets of that population. Other examples of primary prevention include campaigns to encourage the use of seatbelts, correct use of safety seats for infants, fluoridation of water, and smoking cessation. Primary prevention is often supported by national or state government agencies, such as the CDC.

49. D: If a patient with diabetes mellitus, type 1, has been taking insulin injections four times daily and wants to decrease the frequency to twice daily, the best choice of insulin in probably pre-mixed. Pre-mixed insulin combines different proportions of long or intermediate acting and short acting insulins in the same preparations. Pre-mixed insulin is usually administered twice daily and may be appropriate if the available ratio fits the needs of the patient.

50. C: Colorectal cancer screening is usually recommended for patients who are 50-75 years of age. Routine screening options include:

- Fecal occult blood test: Recommended annually.
- Flexible sigmoidoscopy: Recommended every 5 years with fecal occult test every 3 years.
- Colonoscopy: Recommended every 10 years.

If the fecal occult blood test or flexible sigmoidoscopy is positive, then a colonoscopy may be necessary. More frequent colonoscopies may be necessary if risk factors are present, such as ulcerative colitis, family/personal history of colorectal cancer, or colorectal adenomas.

51. B: Tobacco exposure, either from smoking or from inhaling second-hand smoke is a primary risk factor for developing coronary artery or coronary heart disease because nicotine causes vasoconstriction, which in turn increases blood pressure. Additionally, the carbon monoxide that is inhaled decreases the level of oxygen in the blood. Other risk factors include age, male gender (although female's risk increases 10 years after menopause), family history, hypertension, hyperlipidemia, obesity, inactivity, poor diet, and excessive alcohol intake (more than 14/week for males and more than 7/week for females).

52. A: When providing instructions to a patient over the telephone, it's important for the ambulatory care nurse to use plain language and give concise (and clear) instructions. Lengthy explanations can be confusing to the patient, and medical terms should be avoided in favor of plain language whenever possible. While patients should be able to ask questions, interrupting the flow of the instructions to allow questions may cause confusion, so it's better to go through the instructions completely and then to discuss and answer any questions.

53. D: The primary problem that is associated with heart failure is dysfunction of the left ventricle. When peripheral perfusion decreases, such as with hypertension, the kidneys produce renin, which produces a chain reaction resulting in fluid retention and increasing the cardiac workload. The heart loses contractility and blood pools in the ventricles, causing ventricular remodeling and left ventricular dysfunction. The heart compensates with left ventricular hypertrophy, but the blood supply to the enlarged muscle is not adequate, resulting in ischemia.

54. D: Rhinovirus, rubella virus, and influenza have all been documented to spread via airborne transmission. With airborne transmission, small droplets (<5 μm in size) can remain suspended in the air and dispersed widely through air currents or ventilation systems. These viruses can spread when an infected patient coughs or sneezes and can also be spread through direct contact if a person comes in contact with surfaces contaminated with nasal secretions or saliva. This mode of transmission causes these viruses to be highly contagious, infecting about 90% of people who contact the virus and are not immunized.

55. A: A patient who is scheduled for angiograms with contrast should be advised that after administration of the contrast, the patient may feel a sensation of warmth and as though passing urine. These sensations are usually fleeting, and the patient does not usually actually pass urine, but the patient should be encouraged to urinate prior to the procedure. The patient must lie flat for at least 2 hours after the procedure and is usually required to stay in bed for at least a total of four hours.

56. D: In order to be considered copyrighted, material must be original, in a tangible medium (print, recorded, brail, photograph, video) that can be listened to, viewed, read, or understood. The work must be original to the person claiming copyright. The work must also be creative—although the bar is set very low for creativity with almost any effort considered creative. There is no requirement that work carry the copyright symbol or phrase or any statement against fair use. Much material on the internet is copyrighted, so the safest thing to do when linking to other material is to ask permission.

57. A: A patient who has undergone a colonoscopy should be advised to call the physician if the patient experiences persistent abdominal pain, especially if the pain is worsening. Mild abdominal discomfort is common. The patient may experience slight rectal bleeding, but if the bleeding increases or is severe, the patient should notify the physician. Because of irritation caused by the bowel prep done before the procedure, the patient may continue to have one or two loose stools after the procedure. Fever of 100.4°F/38°C or higher should be reported.

58. D: The purpose of completing a hazard vulnerability assessment is to identify gaps in the current all-hazards emergency plan, which all healthcare facilities are required to have. The assessment should assess both human hazards (such as infant abduction, acts of terrorism, civil unrest, mass casualties, hostage situations, bomb threats) and environmental hazards (such as floods, hurricanes, fires, tornados, toxic mold, and earthquakes). The risk is usually classified as not present, low, medium, or high and then the preparedness for the event rated similarly.

59. A: The Rinne test evaluates bone and air conduction and is carried out by holding a vibrating tuning fork on the mastoid bone and measuring the time until the sound ceases. Then the vibrating tuning fork is held at the external ear and the time is measured again until the sound ceases. If there is conductive hearing loss, the sound is heard longer through the bone. If there is sensorineural hearing loss, the sound is heard longer through the air.

60. B: The best source of information about consumer product recalls, such as for car seats, is the Consumer Product Safety Commission, which maintains a database and website. The website contains a list of recall lawsuits that the CPSC has brought in order to seek mandatory recalls. The CPSC provides safety education and descriptions of regulations, laws, and standards. The CPSC is responsible for administering federal laws enacted to protect consumers, such as the Consumer Product Safety Act, the Consumer Product Safety Improvement Plan, the Child Safety Protection Act, and the Poison Prevent Packaging Act.

61. C: OSHA must be notified of a workplace-related death within 8 hours. OSHA is part of the Department of Labor and is charged with ensuring safe, healthful working conditions and setting and enforcing workplace standards. OSHA covers most employers in the private sector, but state and federal safety regulations also generally conform to OSHA standards.

62. B: If a patient became very angry and focused on an unpleasant event (pain during lab testing) and the nurse stated, "It sounds as though that triggered a lot of feelings," this is an example of redirecting. The nurse is attempting to redirect the patient's thoughts and responses from the event itself to feelings about the event, such as feelings of anger, discomfort, frustration, and fear. This shifts the focus back to the patient and encourages the patient to share feelings.

63. B: The ramp function of a CPAP slowly increases the pressure over a period of time to allow the patient to adjust. If the patient feels anxious when wearing the mask, sometimes practicing relaxation exercises can help the patient to fall asleep. In some cases, the mask may be uncomfortable and may be interfering with sleep because it is poorly fitted.

64. A: If a patient states, "I just can't let me parents know that I am pregnant. They will be so upset," a therapeutic response that shows active empathetic listening is: "You feel afraid that your parents won't be supportive." An empathetic response focuses on the feelings of the patient regarding the situation (in this case the pregnancy), based on both verbal and nonverbal communication. Active listening recognizes that everything the patient says and does communicates and that people can perceive the same thing in different ways.

65. C: If an older adult with Alzheimer's begins to exhibit repetitive verbal and physical behavior, such as repeatedly yelling, "Help, help, help, help" and trying to leave, the best way to deal with this behavior is usually with diversion. The ambulatory care nurse should try to engage the patient in an activity, such as looking at pictures in a magazine, or give the patient some item or treat to focus on. Reasoning with a patient with advanced Alzheimer's disease is usually not effective, and restraints often make behavior worse.

66. B: If a patient has a diagnosis of macular degeneration with vision impairment and the ambulatory care nurse must provide information about treatment, the nurse should first ask the patient about the degree of vision impairment and then decide on the best method of presentation. Patients with macular degeneration rarely become completely blind, and the degree of vision impairment may vary widely depending on whether the condition affects one eye or both and whether the macular degeneration is wet or dry.

67. A: If an older patient complains of chronic constipation, which the patient has been self-managing with stimulant laxatives and enemas, and the patient has been advised to stop these treatments, the best initial approach to resolve chronic constipation is increased dietary fiber, with 15 g of fiber per day usually required for effectiveness. The bloating and flatus associated with bran usually subsides within a month of use. If this is not effective, the next approach is a bulk laxative, such as sorbitol, which retains fluid in the bowel and softens the stool.

68. C: If an ambulatory care nurse in a correctional facility is interviewing a prisoner who has been diagnosed with antisocial personality disorder and the patient states that the other healthcare providers have repeatedly failed to treat his health problems, the nurse should attempt to verify the patient's complaints. Patients with antisocial personality disorder tend to be manipulative and deceitful, but no complaints should be dismissed out of hand. Patients with antisocial personality disorder almost never take responsibilities for their problems but blame others and lack insight.

69. B: A group in which all members share a certain trait, such as all patients with heart disease, is classified as a homogeneous group. Although the members may be quite varied (male, female, old, young), they all have the same disorder, and this is the primary focus of the group. The group may be further categorized as *closed* if no further members are allowed or *open* if other members can join.

70. A: A primary obstacle to implementing shared governance at all levels within the nursing department of an ambulatory care center is the differing levels of knowledge and experience. Since most nursing is carried out within a hierarchical structure in which those at the top make decisions, many nurses have little experience making decisions based on research and careful consideration of alternatives. They may have spent little time working in groups or committees. Staff may need ongoing education in order to fully contribute to shared governance.

71. A: If a patient is to receive moderate sedation for an invasive procedure, the patient should respond to verbal commands although sometimes slowly. The patient should have no memory of the procedure or discomfort and should require no assistance with respiratory effort. Cardiovascular function should remain normal. Moderate sedation is often referred to as "conscious sedation" and is the type of sedation commonly used for colonoscopy and various other procedures.

72. D: An injury log must include the location where the incident occurred. All incidents involving needles and sharps must be reported and documented even if no serious injury or illness occurred as a result of the incident. All employees with possible exposure to bloodborne pathogens should receive a hepatitis B vaccination.

73. D: In the initial or orientation phase of a group for which the ambulatory care nurse is serving in the role of leader, the nurse is expected to promote trust and encourage participation. The nurse may describe the group processes and rules and review the overall goals of the group, but it's important not to overwhelm a group with too much information during this initial phase when the members are unsure of whom to trust and how to act.

74. B: If a patient at an urgent care center suffers peritonitis because the triage ambulatory care nurse fails to recognize symptoms of acute appendicitis and requires the patient to wait for three hours before seeing a physician, the type of negligence the nurse is exhibiting is negligent conduct. The nurse provided substandard care that resulted in patient harm. Gross negligence requires that the negligent act be intentional. With contributory negligence, the patient contributes to the harm. With comparative negligence, a percentage of negligence is applied to different individuals who are involved.

75. D: If an ambulatory care nurse has received a verbal order for a medication, but the physician is called away and not available to authenticate the order, Medicare regulations allow the covering physician to do so. Nurse practitioners and physician assistants may not authenticate a physician's orders. Verbal orders must be authenticated in writing or per electronic signature no later than 48 hours after the order was given. Orders received verbally should be designated as "v.o." Verbal orders should be avoided if possible.

76. C: If an older patient complains of urinary frequency and urgency, increasing shortness of breath, pain in the right knee when walking prolonged distances, and chronic constipation, the order of priority (most critical to least) should be:

1. Shortness of breath: Problems with ABCs have priority because they may be life-threatening.
2. Urinary frequency and urgency: This may indicate or increase the risk of infection or renal problems.
3. Chronic constipation: This is an ongoing problem that requires intervention.
4. Pain in right knee: Because this only occurs when walking prolonged distances, this problem has the lowest priority.

77. A: If the ambulatory care nurse believes that the staff of a busy clinic could reduce stress by managing time better, the first place to begin is by completing time logs for a few days because it's difficult to attempt to better manage time until staff members are clear how they are spending their time. Staff members should log every action and the time involved. Once completed, then the time logs can be evaluated to determine where changes may be most effective in saving time.

78. B: If intergroup conflict between two different groups of staff members is causing low morale and increased turnover in the workplace and the ambulatory care nurse wants to help to resolve the conflict, the first step is de-escalation is to identify the conflict boundaries. That is, the nurse needs to determine the parties to the conflict, the causes, and the extent of agreement and disagreement before determining a management strategy. Each group should present its perception of the conflict and its aims.

79. A: If an ambulatory care nurse wants to practice a complementary therapy with patients, the first thing that the nurse should do is to review the state nurse practice act to determine if there are any specific requirements (such as certification) or restrictions. About half of the states allow nurses to practice complementary therapies, but most states require licensure or certification if it is common to the therapy, such as a license to utilize therapeutic massage.

80. B: If a patient advises the ambulatory care nurse in a physician's office that the patient is moving to another state and wants medical records to be sent to a physician who will be assuming care of the patient, the nurse should ask the patient to sign an authorization to release medical records form. This release can indicate whether the patient wants all records or only some records transmitted. While forms may vary somewhat, most forms ask the purpose of the release. In this case, the purpose is for "continuity of medical care."

81. D: The primary problem when screening patients via telephone is lack of nonverbal feedback. The ambulatory care nurse should listen very carefully to the patient's tone of voice and rhythm of speech since the nurse is unable to observe facial reactions or body position. A screening manual with appropriate questions for specific complaints should be available so that staff members screening patients are consistent in asking appropriate questions although additional questions for clarification may be necessary.

82. B: If an ambulatory care center is located near a major highway junction and traffic, braking, and honking sounds are evident in the waiting and examination areas, the best solution may be to provide background music (such as quiet classical music) or white noise (such as a sound like wind) to help to cover the traffic noises and may be soothing. Constant unpleasant noise can be very distracting for both staff and patients and add to stress.

83. A: The Fair Labor Standards Act establishes standards for minimum wage and overtime pay as well as standards for required record keeping and child labor. The Contract Work Hours and Safety Standards Act requires contractors and subcontractors on federal projects worth more than $100,000 to pay overtime of 1.5 times hourly wages for hours more than 40/week and prohibits unsanitary or unsafe working conditions. The McNamara-O'Hara Service Contract Act requires contractors and subcontractors on prime contracts of more than $2,500 to pay workers prevailing wages and benefits, and minimum wage or better on contracts of less than $2,500. The Civil Rights Act (1964) prohibits gender discrimination and sexual harassment by employers.

84. C: If an ambulatory care nurse writes negative comments about their place of employment on a personal social media site that allows public access, such as Facebook, the ambulatory care nurse is likely to be subject to disciplinary action and may even lose employment. Many employers now require that employees agree to make no statements about their place of employment on any social media site, positive or negative, as a safeguard for their reputations.

85. C: These symptoms are consistent with a urinary tract infection, which is not an emergent situation; however, treatment should not be delayed more than a few hours. The triage nurse should encourage the patient to drink adequate fluids.

86. A: While state laws vary somewhat in regard to elder abuse, in virtually all states nurses are considered mandatory reporters, and elder abuse must be reported to the appropriate authorities (usually adult protective services). Older adults are often fearful of reporting the abuser, so the ambulatory care nurse should advise the patient that the nurse is required to report the abuse and should ask the patient if the family member is present in the clinic to determine if a security or police officer is needed.

87. D: Gonorrhea is one of the diseases classified as "standard" by the CDC and requires electronic notification within the next reporting cycle, generally to state public health departments who subsequently report the aggregate results to the CDC. State regulations about communicable diseases may vary somewhat. Diseases that are classified as "immediate, extremely urgent" (such as SARS-associated coronavirus) require reporting by telephone to the CDC within 4 hours and those classified as "immediate, urgent" require reporting within 24 hours.

88. B: If the ambulatory care nurse inadvertently charts a telephone order and medication administration for one patient on the wrong patient's electronic health record (although the right patient got the medication), the correct procedure is to leave the entries and indicate they are errors, following the protocol established by the organization. EHRs should be set up in such a way that information cannot be deleted once it's input. Nurses should carefully review entries to ensure they are correct before finalizing them.

89. C: When educating a patient with mild cognitive impairment (MCI) about wound care, one way to deal with the communication barrier is to break instructions into small steps because carrying out actions that require a number of sequential steps can be very confusing to patients with MCI. The ambulatory care nurse should ask the patient what helps them to learn. Some patients may want to take notes while others may need illustrations or written guides.

90. D: The emergency department staff must deliver the child and placenta and ensure that the patients are stable before transfer in accordance with the Emergency Medical Treatment and Labor Act. This is true even if the facility does not provide obstetric care. All physicians have had some training in obstetrics and should be able to safely deliver an infant. Staff should have training in the assessment of labor.

91. D: If a patient in a clinic has a severe anaphylactic reaction to the Tdap immunization, the event must be reported to the Vaccine Adverse Event Reporting System (VAERS), which is co-sponsored by the CDC and the FDA. Health professionals and manufacturers of vaccines must file reports of specific adverse events. VAERS provides a table that lists vaccines and reportable events and the interval from the time of vaccination. For example, anaphylaxis or anaphylactic shock that occurs within 7 days of Tdap immunization must be reported.

92. A: If a patient scheduled for a liver biopsy at an ambulatory surgery center lists the religion as Jehovah's Witness, the ambulatory care nurse should ask the patient about receiving blood products. Because bleeding is a risk with liver biopsy, the physician should be notified if the patient refuses blood products for religious reasons. In that case, the physician may opt to do the procedure in an acute care facility. While many Jehovah's Witnesses refuse blood products, the nurse should ask rather than assume that is the case.

93. B: If a patient has a foreign body in the eye, and it is visible and does not appear to be imbedded, the best method to remove the foreign body is by gently rolling a moistened cotton-tipped applicator over the foreign body, which should adhere to the applicator. The patient should be in a comfortable supine position. One or two drops of ophthalmic anesthetic should be placed in the eye first to help relieve discomfort and to make it easier to hold the eyelids open.

94. C: While shared governance focuses primarily on empowering nursing, partnership councils focus on members at all levels of an organization and all departments. Rather than one large partnership council, an organization may have a number of partnership councils with one member from each assigned to attend the central council. This prevents the central council from becoming too large to work effectively. Communication flows both vertically and horizontally, and information is shared throughout the organization.

95. A: Before a surgical procedure can be carried out, the ambulatory care nurse should check the patient's health record to ensure that the following documents are in the record: history, physical exam, and signed consent form. The history should contain both current and past medical and social history (including use of alcohol and illicit drugs), lists of medications (prescribed and OTC), lists of allergies, any previous problems with anesthesia or family problems with anesthesia. The physical exam should at the least include assessment of the cardiac status, pulmonary status (including airway patency), and vital signs.

96. A: The purpose of MedWatch, which is provided by the FDA, is to facilitate voluntary reporting of adverse events or sentinel events associated with a medical product (primarily drugs and medical devices). Forms are available on the website, and reports can be made in print, online, or by telephone. MedWatch also receives reports about other products that are regulated by the FDA, including cosmetics, infant foods, and diet supplements. Based on the reports, the FDA may issue safety warnings.

97. C: If a patient requests copies of personal health information contained in an electronic health record at a physician's office, the office should provide the copies the patient has requested within 30 days. If there is a valid reason for a delay, the office may notify the patient in writing of a 30-day delay one time only. If records are stored off-site (such as old paper records), then the office has 60 days to produce copies of the record. However, the records should always be produced as quickly as possible.

98. D: While the federal government has issued some guidelines regarding people's right to have an advance directive, the type of directive needed is determined by state law, so the patient asking about completing an advance directive should be advised to obtain a form that complies with state guidelines. These state forms can be downloaded from the website of the American Bar Association. While advance directives are similar across the states, the state regulations vary on signatures, with some requiring signatures of two witnesses and some requiring a notarized signature.

99. D: When carrying out rapid assessment for triage, the first thing to evaluate is the patient's respirations. If absent, an attempt should be made to open the airway. Those with respirations above 30 bpm should be immediately treated. After respirations, perfusion should be checked by assessing radial pulse and capillary refill. If radial pulse is absent or capillary refill is more than 2 seconds, then immediate attention is required. If perfusion is adequate, then mental status should be evaluated by asking the patient to follow simple commands. If the patient is unable to do so, then immediate care is indicated.

100. A: 2, 4, 1, and 3. If a number of patients arrive simultaneously at an urgent care center, the order in which the patients should be seen is:

1. Severe vaginal bleeding may be life threatening for both the mother and fetus.
2. Stroke victims should be evaluated quickly to determine need for thrombolytic therapy.
3. Fractured femur carries risk of substantial blood loss and fat embolism.
4. The child has relatively mild symptoms so has the lowest priority.

101. C: If a 72-year-old patient complains of increasing fatigue, weakness, dyspnea on exertion, and lack of interest in activities, and the pulse rate increases from 70 to 96, blood pressure from 126/78 to 150/96, and respirations from 18 to 26 three minutes after activity, a likely nursing diagnosis is activity intolerance. The patient must be assessed for cardiovascular or other disorders that could be causing the activity intolerance and imbalance between the supply of oxygen and the demand. The condition can also result from a sedentary lifestyle or long periods of immobility or bedrest.

102. A: When examining and cleansing a wound on a toddler's hand, the best position for the child is in the caregiver's arms in a hug hold. The child is likely to be less frightened and more cooperative if the child feels safe and secure. Whenever possible, if the child requires any type of restraint, the caregiver (often a parent) should be involved because, if the child is restrained by strangers, such as nurses and doctors, the child is likely to scream and fight because of fear.

103. D: The medication reconciliation process should be carried out with a patient in a physician's office at every visit. Before the first visit, the patient should be advised to bring a list of all current medications (including OTC drugs and supplements) at the initial and each subsequent visit and to be sure to include the dosage of each medication. Some physicians may prefer that the patients bring the prescription bottles. Even if the patient does bring a medication list, the nurse should carefully question the patient about medications and supplements.

104. A: If the patient is experiencing shortness of breath or swelling of the tongue or throat, then it is critical that epinephrine, a crash cart, and oxygen be readily available because the patient may be developing anaphylaxis. The site of the sting should be examined to determine if the stinger is still in place so it can be removed, and the extent of swelling should be noted.

105. D: A behavior contract might be an appropriate tool for a patient who repeatedly uses foul language when addressing staff members. Violent patients or those who make threats may need to be reported to the police and may react violently to the suggestion of a behavior contract. Patients must have awareness and reasonably good cognition in order to be a party to a behavior contract, so this usually precludes patients who are intellectually impaired or have dementia (such as a patient with Alzheimer's disease).

106. B: For a patient who takes multiple medications, the food that is most likely one that should be avoided is grapefruit. Grapefruit interferes with an enzyme that is necessary to break down many drugs for elimination, increasing blood levels and risk of adverse reactions. The reaction can last for more than 24 hours. Grapefruit should be avoided with a wide range of medications, including amiodarone, erythromycin, loratadine, lovastatin, fexofenadine, verapamil, simvastatin, and fentanyl transdermal patch.

107. A: For most medications, the primary difference between the brand name drug and the generic version of the drug is the price. Generic drugs tend to be much lower in price than brand name drugs. Some authorities believe that certain brand name medications are superior to the generic, specifically thyroxine products, because of the manner in which drugs are tested for equivalency. Additionally, thyroxine content may vary by more than 10% to the stated dose, and this can pose a problem when dosages need to be precise.

108. B: Low back pain (LBP) is characterized by the duration of symptoms:

- Acute: <6 weeks. The most common form of LBP. Risk factors include lifting, bending, pulling, and stooping. Combining increased activity with sedentary lifestyle may result in LBP.
- Sub-acute: ≥6 weeks to ≤3 months. May indicate underlying pathology, such as spondylitis, osteoporosis, compression fracture, or neoplasm.
- Chronic: ≥3 months to ≤6 months. Similar to sub-acute, but symptoms persist for prolonged period.
- Acute imposed on chronic: Acute flare-ups of pain superimposed on chronic back pain.

109. A: If a non-pregnant patient has had proteinuria ranging from 90 mg/day to 300 mg/day for 3 months, the patient should be referred to a nephrologist for further testing as persistent proteinuria may indicate renal disease. Persistent proteinuria is often associated with an underlying extrarenal disorder, such as hypertension or diabetes. Persistent proteinuria may also be an indication that the patient will eventually develop hypertension or renal insufficiency even if not currently present. Transient proteinuria, such as may occur in an isolated test, is a common occurrence and not considered pathological.

110. A: The MMR (Measles, mumps, and rubella) is from attenuated live viruses. Attenuated viruses are weakened so that they cause the body to produce antibodies against the virus but are too weak to cause disease (although they should be avoided in those with compromised immune systems). The flu vaccine is made with inactivated viruses. Toxoid vaccines, such as diphtheria and tetanus, are made from toxins produced by the virus or bacteria. Some vaccines, such as Hib, are manmade.

111. D: If a patient complains of frequent anxiety and wants to try complementary therapy rather than medications, visualization and relaxation exercises are likely to provide the most relief. Some people also find music therapy relaxation and may use soft music to facilitate relaxation exercises. Patients may be provided a script, guide, or audiotapes to guide them through the visualization and relaxation exercises. Relaxation exercises often involve first tensing and then relaxing muscles, one group at a time while concentrating on breathing.

112. B: The ABN (CMS-R-131) is provided to patients to inform them that Medicare will not cover an item or service. This typically indicates that a supplementary insurance policy will also not cover the item or service. The ABN is given to patients enrolled in Original Medicare, or fee-for-service Medicare. ABNs may also be issued if the patient wants a service or item that is not deemed medically necessary at that time, such as a repeat laboratory test, but is a service or item that is generally covered by Medicare.

113. C: If a 74-year-old patient comes to the ambulatory care center with her daughter, and the daughter beings to describe the patient's problems while the patient remains silent, the best response is to direct questions directly to the patient by name and to observe the response of both the patient and her daughter. There may be a good reason why the daughter is speaking for the patient, such as the patient's cognitive or speech impairment, so asking the daughter to give reasons or to leave the room may be premature and result in animosity.

114. B: Patients who are taking phenytoin for seizure disorders should be advised to have regular dental care because of increased risk of gingival hyperplasia, which can occur both in children and adults and can lead to bleeding, tooth displacement, and periodontal disease. Phenytoin-induced gingival hyperplasia occurs in 15% to 50% of patients taking the medication. Poor oral hygiene is a risk factor, so patients on phenytoin should be educated about the need for regular dental care, brushing and flossing, as well as routine teeth cleaning and examinations by dentists.

115. A: If a patient complains of urinary frequency and urgency, a positive leukocyte esterase dipstick indicates the presence of pyuria and possible urinary tract infection. If symptoms are consistent with infection and the dipstick is positive, it is usually considered diagnostic of UTI without further laboratory testing. The leukocyte esterase dipstick test detects enzymes produced by leukocytes. The same test can be used to screen for infections of amniotic fluid and for gonorrhea.

116. D: If the ambulatory care nurse is teaching a patient to self-administer insulin, and the nurse has instructed the parent to divide each site (abdomen, thigh, and arm) into quadrants, the patient should then be advised to use the same quadrant for one week, rotating about the site in a clockwise fashion. After one week, the next quadrant is used and so on until all four quadrants are completed.

117. B: If a patient comes to the ambulatory care center after experiencing a fall and has a small cut on the forehead, the sign or symptom that may indicate a change in mental status is if the patient repeatedly asks the same question. This suggests that the patient is having a problem with memory, which could indicate a concussion or more serious head injury. The patient should be kept under surveillance and may need to have a head CT if symptoms persist or worsen.

118. B: When discussing home care for a child with the flu and a fever, the ambulatory care nurse should stress that the parent should avoid giving the child aspirin to treat the fever because aspirin can result in Reye's syndrome. Reye's syndrome is a life-threatening disorder that can occur if children with viral infections (especially the flu or chickenpox) take aspirin. Reyes syndrome can cause encephalopathy and liver damage, especially in children between the ages of 4 and 12.

119. C: If when the ambulatory care nurse is screening telephone calls, a patient calls to complain of low back pain, the additional symptoms that represent an emergent situation and should result in the nurse advising the patient to hang up and call 9-1-1 is sudden loss of bowel and bladder control. Pain radiating down the left leg may indicate pressure on the sciatic nerve while fever or burning on urination and frequency may indicate a urinary tract infection. Neither of these conditions are emergent, but appointments should be made as soon as possible.

120. D: If a patient was scheduled for a colonoscopy but misunderstood the directions and did not adequately complete the bowel prep and became very upset when informed the procedure would have to be delayed, the most appropriate nursing diagnosis is "Deficient knowledge." Patients with low literacy may be unable to read or adequately comprehend printed directions resulting in delays and frustration, so the ambulatory care nurse should always review home procedures with patients to ensure they understand.

121. C: When collecting a throat specimen for the rapid strep test, the correct procedure is to swab the back of the throat, including reddened area or pustules. The nurse should ask the patient to say "Ahh" and should use a tongue depressor so the site can be well visualized. The mucous membranes at the back of the throat, the crypts, and the tonsillar areas should all be swabbed. The tongue depressor should be held in place until the swab is withdrawn from the mouth.

122. D: If the ambulatory care nurse is to administer eye drops to a patient, but drainage and crusts are evident along the eyelid margins and inner canthus, the first step is to soak the crusts with a warm damp cloth or cotton ball for a few minutes and then wipe clean from the inner canthus to the outer. Scrubbing back and forth or irrigating should be avoided because the crusts and drainage may contain pathogenic organisms.

123. C: Following a surgical procedure at an ambulatory surgery center, if the patient must be taught to use a flow-oriented incentive spirometer, unlicensed assistive personnel (UAP) can teach the skill of using the spirometer to the patient. However, UAP cannot monitor the patient's frequency of use, assess the patient's use of the spirometer to ensure it is used correctly, or evaluate the patient's response to the use of the spirometer because these are nursing skills.

124. C: When fitting a patient for crutches, measure from 2 inches below the axilla to 6 inches in front of the patient. This allows the patient to advance the crutches and step without having to lean forward, because leaning forward could destabilize the patient and cause a fall. Another option is to measure from the anterior axillary fold to the sole of the foot. The patient should be able to comfortably grasp the handpiece when standing up straight, supported by the crutches, with the arms flexed at 20-30 degrees, because this provides room for extension when the patient moves the crutches forward.

125. C: Low-income patients may be eligible for the FCC's Lifeline service, which provides a $9.25 subsidy toward wired or wireless telephone service or discounted broadband service. The service is intended for low-income individuals whose income is at or below 135% of the federal poverty level. Patients who are eligible for a number of different programs are also eligible: Federal Public Housing, Section 8, Supplemental Nutrition Assistance Program, Medicaid, SSI, TANF, National School lunch program, and Low-Income Home Energy Assistance Program. Additionally, those residing on tribal lands and participating in federal or state assistance programs are eligible.

126. A: As a case manager for a stroke patient who has been discharged home but is having difficulty preparing foods because of residual right-sided weakness, the most appropriate referral is to an occupational therapist. Occupational therapists can help the patient with exercises to increase strength in the right hand and can also show the patient how to compensate for the right-sided weakness and how to use assistive devices in order to cook safely.

127. D: All staff members in a healthcare facility must receive education regarding compliance issues, although the education may vary depending on the position and responsibilities. The compliance program must have written policies and procedures that include standards of conduct. The written policies and procedures should be provided to all members of the organization and should be reviewed and updated routinely, at least on an annual basis. Standards of compliance should be monitored and enforced.

128. D: A patient who has received an anesthetic agent at an ambulatory surgery center must be supervised by a responsible adult following the procedure for at least 12-24 hours, depending on the patient's general condition, type of surgery, and type of anesthesia. Patients should be advised of the need for supervision prior to the procedure and should not be discharged until a responsible person is present. Patients should not be discharged per taxi or allowed to drive themselves home.

129. A: The primary purpose of a "time out" prior to beginning a surgical procedure is to confirm the correct patient (checking two IDs), the correct procedure, and the correct surgical markings in order to prevent surgical error. The surgery should not proceed until all questions have been answered and concerns addressed. If special equipment, prosthetics, or other implants are needed for the surgical procedure, then their presence should be confirmed as well.

130. B: The emergency power source for the ambulatory surgery center should be able to operate the lighting and equipment in operating rooms for a period of at least two hours as this duration should be sufficient to complete most procedures carried out in ASCs. Emergency power sources should be available for all operating rooms and should be up and running within 30 seconds if the power fails. Lighting should be sufficient in all corridors to allow safe passage.

131. C: The purpose of the Caffeine Halothane Contracture Test is to determine if a patient will exhibit malignant hyperthermia, an inherited condition in which the patient develops a very high body temperature and muscle contracture after exposure to inhalational anesthesia and/or succinylcholine. The Caffeine Halothane Contracture Test is available at only 4 sites in the United States, but patients at risk should be referred for testing, which requires a muscle biopsy.

132. A: A decreased TSH (produced by the pituitary gland) and decreased free T4 (produced by the thyroid gland) indicate hypothyroidism associated with disease of the pituitary gland. When levels of free T4 fall, the normal pituitary gland produces TSH, which stimulates the thyroid gland to produce free T4, but if the pituitary gland is not producing adequate TSH to stimulate the thyroid gland, then both levels fall. If the hypothyroidism results from disease of the thyroid gland, then the TSH level elevates and the free T4 level decreases.

133. C: If the ambulatory care nurse is to collect a wound specimen for culture and sensitivities, the correct procedure is to collect the specimen from inside the wound after applying an antiseptic to the tissue about the wound and then allowing the swab to saturate with discharge. The outer edges of the wound should be avoided when removing the swab as the surface of the skin may contain bacteria that can contaminate the specimen.

134. D: If a patient is scheduled for an abdominal CT with IV contrast, it is important to ask the patient about allergies to iodine, especially previous reactions to IV contrast, because the IV contrast is iodine-based. While there is some concern that those who are allergic to shellfish may have cross-reactivity, studies indicate that about 85% of patients allergic to shellfish tolerate the IV contrast material without an allergic response, about the same percentage as those allergic to anything else.

135. C: A patient scheduled for cardiac stress testing should be advised to avoid caffeine for 12 hours before the test because it is a stimulant and can affect heart rate. Patients are usually advised to avoid all foods and drinks except water for 4 hours before the test to prevent nausea and vomiting. Patients who will walk on the treadmill should be advised to wear comfortable loose-fitting clothing and comfortable walking shoes.

136. A: The NIOSH Hierarchy of Controls is as follows:

- **Elimination**: Eliminate the hazard and change the practice; this is the most effective intervention but also the most expensive or difficult to achieve.
- **Substitution**: Use a different piece of equipment or process or a different chemical.
- **Engineering controls**: Use shields, barriers, ventilation hoods, guardrails, soundproofing, air conditioning, and equipment guards.
- **Administrative controls**: Provide signage, training, an adjusted work schedule, and rest periods.
- **Personal protective equipment**: Helmets, safety glasses, gloves, gowns, respirators, and face shields. This is the least effective control and often indicates an inability to carry out adequate controls at a higher level.

137. B: The ethnic group that has the highest prevalence of asthmas is African Americans, especially among children, with the rate in African American children almost 60% higher than in Caucasian children. Rates are also high among Native Americans and Puerto Ricans. Because of the disparity in rates of asthma, children in these ethnic groups should be routinely screened for signs of asthma and preventive treatment prescribed as indicated and parents/caregivers educated about environmental triggers.

138. C: Females should be screened for cervical cancer every 3 years from ages 21-65 although if females are sexually active at an earlier age, some physicians may recommend earlier initial screening. In some cases, screening every 5 years between ages 30 and 65 may be recommended with cytology and HPV testing. The rates of cervical cancer should begin to fall if the HPV vaccination becomes widely administered to both boys and girls.

139. B: Overweight and obesity are categorized according to BMI:

- 18.5-24.9: Desirable
- 25-29.9: Overweight
- 30-34.9: Class I obesity
- 35-39.9: Class II obesity
- Over 40: Class III obesity (severe)

Patients are usually defined as obese if their weight is 120% of that desired or the percent of body fat is more than 25% for males and more than 33% for females (females have a greater percentage of body fat than males).

140. B: Up to 15% of children from ages 4-14 experience growing pains. Usually, the child is free of pain in the morning but develops pain later in the day. Treatment typically includes massage, warm compresses, and stretching exercises as well as acetaminophen or ibuprofen for discomfort.

141. C: In this situation, the spouse whose insurance is primary is the spouse whose birthday comes first in the year (the birthday rule). Coordination of benefits comprises the rules that insurance companies use to ensure that no healthcare provider receives more than 100% of the charges submitted for services rendered. State regulations regarding coordination of benefits may vary somewhat, and some insurance policies have no coordination of benefits rules.

142. D: If a patient is receiving methotrexate as a chemotherapeutic agent, the antidote that may be co-administered to decrease adverse effects of methotrexate is leucovorin calcium (a folic acid analog), which serves to protect healthy cells. Leucovorin calcium may also be used to counteract an overdose of methotrexate. Leucovorin is taken orally. Leucovorin may cause various adverse effects, including diarrhea, skin rash, urticaria, dyspnea, and dysphagia.

143. B: If a patient states she plans to take St. John's Wort for mild depression rather than an SSRI, the ambulatory care nurse should carefully review the patient's list of medications. While St. John's Wort has been shown to be effective for some patients for mild depression, it interacts negatively with many medications, in many cases decreasing the effectiveness of the drugs (such as oral contraceptives and digoxin). St. John's Wort should be avoided during pregnancy.

144. A: If a patient comes to the ambulatory care centers complaining of chest pain and shortness of breath, the first action of the ambulatory care nurse should be to take the patient by wheelchair to an examination room with a crash cart/tray nearby in the event the patient experiences a cardiac arrest. Then, the patient should be questioned further and vital signs, oxygen saturation level, and ECG taken. Oxygen may be administered if necessary to relieve dyspnea, depending on oxygen saturation level.

145. C: If a patient faints while awaiting an examination at an ambulatory care center and complains of feeling very weak and faint after regaining consciousness, the ambulatory nurse should place the patient in Trendelenburg position. The nurse should take the patient's vital signs and question the patient about previous history of fainting. The nurse should document events that occurred before the fainting episode and note the duration that the patient was unconscious. Any heart irregularities, shortness of breath, or injuries incurred should be documented.

146. D: Discharge from the post-anesthesia care unit (PACU) requires a score of 9-10. Five different items are assessed, each scored on a scale of 0-2: activity (ability to move), respiration, circulation (blood pressure, skin color), consciousness (awake/arousable), and oxygenation.

147. B: If a patient comes to the ambulatory care center 10 minutes after being stung by a bee, and the patient is developing rapid generalized edema and shortness of breath, the treatment that the nurse anticipates is epinephrine as these symptoms may be indications that the patient is developing anaphylaxis. A crash cart/tray should be available. Hypersensitivity reactions usually occur within an hour of a sting although the reaction can be delayed in some patients.

148. B: Following a minor surgical procedure for which the patient received moderate ("conscious") sedation, the patient should expect to be discharged after 1-2 hours. Patients usually are alert and responsive within a short period after sedation is discontinued although they may remain slightly drowsy. The patient should be discharged in a wheelchair to a waiting vehicle. Patients should not drive and should have a responsible adult in attendance for 12-24 hours after the procedure.

149. A: If, following a surgical procedure in which the patient received moderate sedation, the patient's blood pressure drops to 85/48 from a preoperative level of 126/84, the initial response is usually to increase intravenous fluids. The patient should be thoroughly assessed to determine if the cause is hypovolemia or opioids. Hypotension is a common occurrence in the postoperative period and is usually transient. Naloxone may be indicated if the patient's hypotension is associated with opioid administration.

150. D: When assessing key performance measures as part of the ambulatory care process improvement assessment, one of the key performance measures for access to care is the average telephone wait time, the telephone abandonment rate, and total calls per agent. Other key performance measures for access to care include the availability of appointment times, the number and frequency of rescheduled appointments, wait time in the waiting room and the exam room, the appointment cancellation rate, consult and referral request turnaround, and availability of open appointment times for walk-in or urgent care patients.

Practice Test #2

1. If two staff members in an ambulatory care center have an ongoing conflict because of personality issues and this conflict is interfering with their work, the best recourse is likely to:

a. Sit both parties down and attempt conflict resolution.
b. Ensure that the employees are scheduled to work at different times.
c. Fire the employee that is most at fault.
d. Fire both employees for unprofessional conduct.

2. If a patient with a history of atrial fibrillation takes warfarin as an anticoagulant, the patient's international normalized ratio (INR) should usually remain between:

a. 1 and 2
b. 2 and 3
c. 3 and 4
d. 4 and 5

3. The temperature in operating rooms is usually maintained at:

a. 60 °F (16 °C) to 65 °F (18 °C)
b. 65 °F (18 °C) to 68 °F (20 °C)
c. 68 °F (20 °C) to 73 °F (23 °C)
d. 70 °F (21 °C) to 76 °F (24 °C)

4. Which of the following federal agencies is responsible for regulating medical devices, such as respirators, to ensure that they are safe to use?

a. EPA
b. OSHA
c. Centers for Disease Control and Prevention
d. Food and Drug Administration

5. The primary purpose of risk management is to:

a. Define professional liability and minimize risks.
b. Negotiate settlements for malpractice and negligence.
c. Educate staff about risks.
d. Reduce costs.

6. For a 50-year-old patient whose mammogram shows an abnormal mass in the right breast, the diagnostic procedure of choice is generally a(n):

a. Fine-needle aspiration cytology
b. Large-core needle biopsy
c. Open biopsy
d. Stereotactic biopsy

7. Which of the following is a violation of HIPAA regulations?

a. A nurse shares information about a minor patient to the legal guardian.
b. A nurse allows a patient to see her own laboratory reports.
c. The organization uses de-identified health information for research.
d. A nurse shares personal information about a patient with a nurse not assigned to that patient.

8. The primary mode of action of combined oral contraceptives is:

a. Prevention of implantation
b. Sloughing of implanted cells
c. Suppression of ovulation
d. Spermicidal activity

9. Which of the following is NOT indicative of respiratory abnormality?

a. Rhonchi
b. Vesicular breath sounds
c. Rales
d. Wheezing

10. If an entity, such as an ambulatory care center, experienced a HIPAA violation because of willful neglect of HIPAA rules, but the entity tried to correct the violation (a category 3 violation), what type of fine might be imposed?

a. $100 to $50,000 per episode
b. $10,000 to $50,000 per episode
c. $50,000 per episode
d. $50,000 to $100,000 per episode

11. When reviewing a patient's urinalysis, the ambulatory care nurse notes the presence of white cell casts. This finding is commonly found with:

a. Diuretic therapy
b. Glomerulonephritis
c. Pyelonephritis
d. Acute tubular necrosis

12. If a patient is taking lithium to control bipolar disorder, what electrolyte should be routinely monitored?

a. Potassium
b. Magnesium
c. Calcium
d. Sodium

13. The most common reasons for incident reports are:

a. Patient abuse and neglect
b. Wrong-site surgical procedures
c. Medication errors and falls
d. Equipment malfunctions

14. A patient is prescribed sulfasalazine for treatment of rheumatoid arthritis. Patient teaching should include:

a. The importance of drinking extra fluids
b. The need to take an antacid with the medication
c. The importance of storing the medication in the refrigerator
d. The need to make up a missed dose by taking a double dose

15. If learning takes place outside the formal classroom, with materials provided or recommended by an instructor, the educational model is:

a. Collaborative
b. Project based
c. Goal focused
d. Guided focus

16. A mother bringing her teenager into the ambulatory clinic is concerned that the child has a fruity odor to her breath and is sleepy more than usual. The child seems to skip meals and become nauseated frequently. What on-site, quick laboratory test may give an initial idea about what might be causing the fruity breath and sleepiness?

a. Urine dipstick and HbA1c
b. Urine dipstick and blood glucose
c. Blood glucose only
d. HbA1c only

17. A patient who is diagnosed with Huntington's disease (an autosomal-dominant disorder) is concerned about passing the mutated gene on to his children. What is the percentage chance of passing the disorder to each child?

a. 25%
b. 50%
c. 75%
d. 100%

18. According to Kolb's learning styles inventory, a person who prefers to learn through a combination of concrete experience and active experimentation, solves problems through trial and error, and tends to complete tasks, is classified as:

a. Accommodative
b. Assimilative
c. Divergent
d. Convergent

19. An adult male presents to the ambulatory care setting with a 24-hour history of wheezing, coughing, and shortness of breath. What would be the most appropriate initial procedure that he may require from the nurse in this setting?

a. Blood glucose monitoring
b. Urine dipstick
c. Steroid injection
d. A nebulizer treatment

20. A patient abruptly developed right-sided facial paresis that worsened over 24 hours, as well as hyperacusis (sensitivity to everyday sounds) and an impaired sense of taste. These signs and symptoms are characteristic of:

a. Stroke
b. Parkinson's disease
c. Bell's palsy
d. Myasthenia gravis

21. When training staff for disaster preparedness, it is most important that staff members understand:

a. The local risk for disasters
b. Their roles and responsibilities during a disaster
c. What backup systems are available
d. What supplies will be available

22. A patient is receiving chemotherapeutic agents that can cause myelosuppression. The patient's absolute neutrophil count (ANC) is 700, which indicates:

a. A normal risk for infection
b. A slight risk of infection
c. A significant risk of infection
d. A severe risk of infection

23. The three stages of chemotherapy for leukemia are:

a. Initiation, compliance, and recovery
b. Acute, current, and chronic
c. Induction, compliance, and recovery
d. Induction, consolidation, and maintenance

24. According to the Institute for Healthcare Improvement, patient safety rounds should be conducted at least every:

a. Day
b. 3 days
c. Week
d. Month

25. A female patient who is positive for the BRCA1 and BRCA2 mutations is at risk of breast cancer and:

a. Ovarian cancer
b. Leukemia
c. Lung cancer
d. Renal carcinoma

26. If a serious adverse event occurs, the initial response should include a:

a. Disciplinary hearing
b. Program audit
c. Failure mode and effects analysis
d. Root cause analysis (RCA)

27. When irrigating a wound with normal saline, the irrigation pressure should typically range from:

a. 1-5 psi
b. 5-10 psi
c. 10-15 psi
d. 20-25 psi

28. Which of the following statements is true regarding sterilization and disinfection?

a. Sterilization is the elimination of most pathogenic bacteria/microorganisms (except spores) from objects through the use of chemicals.
b. The purpose of sterilization and disinfection is to prevent transmission of disease from one patient to the next.
c. Disinfection is the destruction of all microorganisms on a surface through both chemical and physical mechanisms.
d. Sterilization and disinfection are regulated by the Joint Commission.

29. The primary principle of quality process improvement is that improvement:

a. Can be accomplished through small, incremental steps
b. Must be part of a master plan
c. Requires all staff members to participate
d. Takes time and continual effort

30. A patient spilled hot wax on her hands, resulting in sloughing of the dermis with large blisters and red, weeping exposed tissue, as well as much pain. This type of burn is classified as:

a. First-degree
b. Second-degree
c. Third-degree
d. Fourth-degree

31. If the ambulatory care nurse allows a parent to accompany a child into the surgical area while the child receives an anesthetic in order to reduce the child's anxiety, this is an example of:

a. Empowerment
b. Healthcare advocacy
c. Patient advocacy
d. Healthcare navigation

32. A patient who has been receiving radiation for cancer treatment has developed erythema and slight edema at the radiation site, as well as sensations of itching and burning. What stage of irradiation damage has occurred?

a. Stage I
b. Stage II
c. Stage III
d. Stage IV

33. Which of the following is an example of therapeutic communication?

a. "Don't worry, I'm sure everything will be all right."
b. "I see that you are upset."
c. "You should consider further treatments."
d. "Oh my goodness, why are you so upset?"

34. With urine dipstick testing, which of the following positive results is likely an indication of a urinary tract infection?

a. Nitrites
b. Bilirubin
c. Ketones
d. Protein

35. In a leadership role, an effective strategy for giving feedback about an issue to another nurse includes:

a. Using judgmental statements
b. Focusing on negative feedback
c. Being objective and specific about the issue
d. Delaying feedback until a convenient time

36. If a person has been drinking alcohol, how long does it usually take for the alcohol to be absorbed into the bloodstream?

a. 10 minutes
b. 30 minutes
c. 60 minutes
d. 90 minutes

37. What approach to conflict resolution is exemplified by trying to find a solution that works for everyone using a step-by-step approach?

a. Problem solving
b. Collaborating
c. Negotiating
d. Compromising

38. Cocaine increases levels of which neurotransmitter?

a. Acetylcholine
b. Epinephrine
c. Gamma-aminobutyric acid
d. Dopamine

39. Place of Service (POS) Codes are used throughout the healthcare industry to:

a. Indicate the town or city in which a service occurred.
b. Indicate the setting where a service occurred.
c. Indicate the area of the country in which the service occurred.
d. Indicate the state in which the service occurred.

40. Screening for bone mineral density with a dual-energy x-ray absorptiometry (DEXA) scan is recommended by the US Preventive Services Task Force for:

a. All women 50 and older
b. All women 60 and older
c. All men and women 60 and older
d. All women 65 and older

41. The nurse practicing in an ambulatory care setting understands that performance improvement becomes part of the responsibility of the healthcare team. Which item would be a performance improvement indicator for an ambulatory care facility and the healthcare team?

a. Payroll
b. Critical pathways
c. Tracer methodology
d. Cost-benefit analysis

42. The first-line drug of choice for treatment of type 2 diabetes mellitus is:

a. A biguanide (e.g., metformin)
b. A sulfonylurea (e.g., glipizide)
c. A meglitinide analog (e.g., repaglinide)
d. A glucagon-like peptide-1 receptor agonist (e.g., semaglutide)

43. Which of the following is generally a nonbillable service under Medicare?

a. Annual flu shot
b. Preventive examination (age >65)
c. A1c testing (for diabetics)
d. Hearing examination to prescribe a hearing aid

44. If a patient has developed herpes zoster (shingles), treatment with antivirals should begin within:

a. 24 hours
b. 48 hours
c. 72 hours
d. 96 hours

45. Approximately what percentage of modifiable contributors to healthy outcomes is attributed to social determinants of health?

a. 90% to 100%
b. 80% to 90%
c. 40% to 50%
d. 20% to 30%

46. The recommended treatment for chlamydial infection (*Chlamydia trachomatis*) for adolescents and adults is:

a. Ceftriaxone 500 mg intramuscularly (IM)
b. Metronidazole 500 mg twice a day (BID) for 7 days
c. Benzathine penicillin G, 2.4 million units IM
d. Doxycycline 100 mg orally BID for 7 days

47. Which population is most vulnerable to food insecurity?

a. Older adults
b. Adults
c. Children
d. Immigrants

48. A patient complains of nasal stuffiness, an impaired sense of smell, headache, and severe throbbing pain around the left eye. These symptoms are consistent with:

a. Acute sinusitis
b. COVID-19
c. Optic neuritis
d. An infected tooth

49. A patient is to receive fluorouracil (5-FU) as part of the treatment for colorectal cancer. The patient should be advised to immediately report:

a. Fatigue and general malaise
b. Nausea
c. Diarrhea
d. Bleeding gums

50. When caring for incarcerated patients, the health problem that is most prevalent is:

a. Substance abuse
b. Infectious diseases
c. Sexually transmitted diseases
d. Anxiety and depression

51. A patient with type 1 diabetes mellitus takes insulin glargine once daily in the evening and is to add rapid-acting insulin lispro before each meal to achieve better blood sugar control. The patient should be advised to eat the meals within:

a. 5 minutes of the insulin lispro
b. 15 minutes of the insulin lispro
c. 30 minutes of the insulin lispro
d. 60 minutes of the insulin lispro

52. If addressing a patient who is deaf but who is able to read lips, the ambulatory care nurse should:

a. Face the patient at 3-6 feet in distance away from the patient.
b. Speak very slowly and in an exaggerated fashion.
c. Avoid facial expressions while speaking.
d. Stand within 2-3 feet of the patient.

53. When irrigating the ear of an adult, the ambulatory care nurse should:

a. Maintain the normal position of the ear.
b. Pull the pinna down and forward.
c. Pull the pinna down and back.
d. Pull the pinna up and back.

54. When communicating with a patient who has global aphasia, the best way to communicate is through:

a. Speaking
b. Diagrams, gestures, and picture charts
c. Reading and writing
d. Gestures only

55. If a patient is receiving moderate (conscious) sedation, the ambulatory care nurse expects that the patient:

a. Will exhibit purposeful response to verbal/tactile stimuli
b. May need an airway intervention
c. Will exhibit impaired spontaneous ventilation
d. Will have a memory of the procedure

56. Microsocial advocacy is aimed at:

a. The patient and family
b. Service organizations
c. The community populations
d. Global populations

57. For blood flow through a vascular access for dialysis, what is the threshold that indicates dysfunction?

a. <300 mL per minute
b. <500 mL per minute
c. <700 mL per minute
d. <100 mL per minute

58. If a patient is to begin peritoneal dialysis, the catheter should be inserted:

a. 1 week before initiation of the treatment
b. 2 weeks before initiation of the treatment
c. 3 weeks before initiation of the treatment
d. 2 months before initiation of the treatment

59. The primary difference between accreditation and certification is that:

a. Certification applies to an entire organization and accreditation applies to programs within the organization.
b. Accreditation applies to an entire organization and certification applies to programs within the organization.
c. Accreditation and certification are mutually exclusive so only one is necessary.
d. Accreditation requires preparation whereas certification only requires application.

60. According to the Substance Abuse and Mental Health Services Administration (SAMHSA), the three E's of trauma are:

a. Events, experiences, and effects
b. Evaluate, educate, and empower
c. Encounter, encourage, and empower
d. Empathy, education, and empowerment

61. Medicare C refers to:

a. Coverage for inpatient care
b. Coverage for outpatient care
c. Coverage for prescription drugs
d. Medicare Advantage plans

62. An adolescent comes to an urgent care center with a nasal fracture after being hit in the face with a hard ball. The ambulatory care nurse notes clear nasal discharge, which may represent a(n):

a. Normal response to swelling
b. Sinus infection
c. Leakage of cerebrospinal fluid
d. Anxiety response

63. Which type of text message to a patient requires prior written consent?

a. Billing notice
b. Appointment reminder
c. Laboratory results
d. Medical instructions

64. Following a dental avulsion, the tooth must be reimplanted within:

a. 60 minutes
b. 1-2 hours
c. 2-4 hours
d. 4-6 hours

65. Under the Payne-Martin Classification System for Skin Tears, a partial-thickness flap skin tear that leaves enough avulsed skin to adequately cover the wound would be classified as:

a. Category I
b. Category II
c. Category III
d. Category IV

66. Which of the following indicates the highest level of patient engagement in the healthcare process?

a. The patient receives information about his or her diagnosis.
b. The patient receives direct treatment with consent.
c. The patient's preferences and best practices guide treatment.
d. The patient is asked about preferences when developing treatment plan.

67. A patient has developed fever, chills, and general muscle and joint aches as well as a large area of erythema migrans (bull's-eye rash) on the upper back, indicating that the patient is at risk for:

a. Chagas disease
b. Mononucleosis
c. *Staphylococcus* infection
d. Lyme disease

68. A 40-year-old patient with a history of chronic illness is alert and responsive, but he brings a bag of medications to an office visit and cannot name the medications or explain why he is taking them. The ambulatory care nurse should suspect that the reason for this is:

a. Impaired functional status
b. Low health literacy
c. Impaired cognitive ability
d. Lack of interest

69. If a patient with human immunodeficiency virus (HIV) is routinely monitored with CD4 counts, what CD4 count indicates a change in diagnosis to acquired immunodeficiency syndrome (AIDS)?

a. < 500 cells/mm^3
b. < 400 cells/mm^3
c. < 300 cells/mm^3
d. < 200 cells/mm^3

70. A patient is prescribed a transcutaneous electrical nerve stimulation (TENS) device to relieve chronic low back pain. To ensure that the correct settings are achieved, the ambulatory care nurse should:

a. Review the recommended settings and set the device accordingly.
b. Ask the physician for the specific settings.
c. Use the lowest settings for the first week and then increase the settings.
d. Adjust the settings slowly until the patient experiences relief.

71. Considering shared decision-making, which of the following is an example of choice talk?

a. The patient and healthcare provider evaluate the choice of treatment.
b. The patient and healthcare provider make decisions based on patient preferences and input.
c. The healthcare provider provides a detailed explanation of options for treatment.
d. The healthcare provider provides an overview of options for treatment.

72. In conditions of high heat (>100 °F), which is the only mechanism of heat dissipation that is effective?

a. Conduction
b. Convection
c. Evaporation
d. Radiation

73. If an ambulatory care nurse works in an outreach clinic with an immigrant patient population that is primarily Spanish speaking, the most effective strategy in building rapport is to:

a. Study medical Spanish.
b. Have materials printed in Spanish.
c. Have an interpreter/translator available.
d. Provide patient information about available English classes.

74. A patient reports a small scratch from a bat that she caught to remove it from her house. The emergent treatment must include:

a. An antibiotic
b. A rabies vaccine
c. An antiviral
d. Topical mupirocin

75. Which of the following skin lesions is precancerous?

a. Acrochordons (skin tags)
b. Cherry angiomas
c. Actinic keratosis
d. Seborrheic keratosis

76. A patient has Alzheimer's disease with middle-stage dementia and communication problems. He has been rubbing his head and saying, "Hurt, hurt." Which is the most appropriate question?

a. "Could you describe your headache for me?"
b. "Do you have a bad headache?"
c. "On a scale of 1-10, how would you rate your headache?"
d. "What part of your head hurts the most?"

77. According to the National Institutes of Health, females age 51 and older and males older than age 70 should consume how many milligrams of calcium daily?

a. 600 mg
b. 800 mg
c. 1,000 mg
d. 1,200 mg

78. Which is the rescue treatment of choice for an acute asthma attack?

a. Short-acting beta 2-agonist (SABA)
b. Long-acting beta 2-agonist (LABA)
c. Low-dose inhaled corticosteroid (ICS)
d. Leukotriene receptor antagonist (LTRA)

79. A patient with a long history of alcoholism and cirrhosis of the liver presents with increasing confusion, ataxia, and impaired vision. The ambulatory care nurse recognizes that these signs are likely indicative of:

a. Alzheimer's disease
b. Parkinson's disease
c. Stroke
d. Wernicke-Korsakoff syndrome

80. If a patient has trigeminal neuralgia affecting the right side of the face, the ambulatory care nurse should advise the patient to:

a. Avoid chewing on the affected side.
b. Ingest only liquids to avoid chewing.
c. Sip iced liquids when pain occurs.
d. Use mouthwash instead of brushing the teeth.

81. The five A's for developing interventions based on the needs of the individual are ask, advise, assess, assist, and:

a. Accept
b. Achieve
c. Adopt
d. Arrange

82. The most common use of ambulatory care nurses in the coordination of care is:

a. Short-term management of patients with acute illness
b. Long-term management of patients with chronic illness
c. Outreach to individuals to encourage compliance with treatment
d. Managing underserved patient populations

83. The revenue cycle of a patient begins with the patient's admission and ends with:

a. Completed billing
b. Completed patient care
c. Receipt of revenue
d. The end of the year

84. Which of the following symptoms are most common to Parkinson's disease?

a. Tremor, bradykinesia, muscle rigidity, shuffling gait, and micrographia
b. Eyelid drooping, diplopia, dysphagia, muscle weakness, and impaired speaking
c. Tremor, vision impairment, weakness of one or more limbs, and slurred speech
d. Waddling gait, muscle pain/stiffness, and impaired ability to rise from sitting or lying

85. The most common transition that the ambulatory care nurse helps to manage is the:

a. Transition from the emergency department or urgent care to an acute hospital
b. Transition from the home environment to extended care
c. Transition from ambulatory care to an acute hospital
d. Transition from an acute hospital to ambulatory care

86. A 60-year-old patient has experienced repeated skin infections, including abscesses and boils as well as fungal infections under the breasts and in other skin folds. The patient should be assessed for:

a. HIV
b. Diabetes mellitus
c. Parasites
d. Anemia

87. An ambulatory care nurse is licensed in two states. The nurse is providing telehealth services for a physician's office to a patient in the state in which the nurse does not reside. The physician lives in a third state. The nurse must provide services in accordance with:

a. The nurse practice act of the state in which the patient resides
b. The nurse practice act of the state in which the nurse resides
c. Either nurse practice act because the nurse is licensed in both states
d. The nurse practice act in the third state, in which the physician resides

88. If a patient has not been responsive to education about changing unhealthy behavior and the ambulatory care nurse is using the five R strategy, the first step is to:

a. Outline all of the risks associated with continuing the unhealthy behavior.
b. List and describe the rewards associated with changing the behavior.
c. Discuss the relevance for the individual of making changes.
d. Identify and discuss roadblocks to the individual's changing behavior.

89. When assessing a patient via telehealth, which of the following is an objective finding?

a. The patient reports a severe cough.
b. The patient reports a blood pressure reading of 180/96 on their home blood pressure cuff.
c. The patient complains of feeling very feverish.
d. All findings via telehealth are subjective.

90. If an ambulatory care nurse in the PACU of an ambulatory surgery center leaves a patient in the PACU unattended without transferring the care of the patient to another nurse, this is an example of:

a. Nursing abandonment
b. Gross negligence
c. Malpractice
d. Abuse

91. The primary purpose of using decision support tools (DSTs) (protocols, algorithms, and guidelines) during telehealth visits is to:

a. Control the process of care.
b. Prevent errors in judgment.
c. Supplement the nurse's knowledge.
d. Promote positive outcomes.

92. Fatal accidents at the workplace or accidents that result in hospitalization of three or more staff members must be reported to OSHA within:

a. 4 hours
b. 8 hours
c. 12 hours
d. 24 hours

93. The purpose of the enhanced Nurse Licensure Compact (eNLC) is to:

a. Speed the process of licensure applications in multiple states.
b. Prevent nurses who lost their nursing licenses from gaining licensure in another state.
c. Share disciplinary information among boards of nursing in multiple states.
d. Provide a multistate license to nurses.

94. When developing a nurse residency program in order to increase retention of newly licensed RNs in an ambulatory care center, the ideal duration of the program is:

a. 3-6 months
b. 6 months
c. 6-9 months
d. 9-12 months

95. A key principle of telehealth triage is to:

a. Assume that frequent contacts are unnecessary.
b. Consider every call life-threatening.
c. Depend on decision support tools.
d. Accept individual self-diagnosis.

96. When creating a series of educational posters for patients utilizing three different colors, the primary color should comprise about:

a. 40% of the display
b. 50% of the display
c. 70% of the display
d. 90% of the display

97. Under the patient-centered medical home model of providing care, the gold standard for care delivery is:

a. Functional care
b. Telehealthcare
c. Team-based care
d. Modular care

98. The vaccine Shingrix, which protects against herpes zoster, is recommended for all healthy adults ages:

a. 65 and older
b. 60 and older
c. 55 and older
d. 50 and older

99. Following cataract surgery, which of the following activities is generally prohibited for up to 4-6 weeks?

a. Jogging
b. Weight lifting
c. Yoga
d. Golf

100. The primary purpose of harm-reduction principles in nursing is to:

a. Prevent injuries, such as falls, in patients.
b. Decrease the incidence of violence and aggressive behavior.
c. Prevent adverse effects associated with treatments.
d. Decrease the negative effects of unhealthy behaviors.

101. If a patient was stung by a bee and the stinger remains in the skin, the best way to remove the stinger is to:

a. Scrape a sharp instrument over the skin.
b. Use tweezers to remove the stinger.
c. Squeeze the tissue around the stinger.
d. Soak the area in warm, soapy water.

102. Approximately what percentage of patients who experience a transient ischemic attack (TIA) will have a stroke within a year of the TIA?

a. 25%
b. 33%
c. 50%
d. 66%

103. If using constraint-induced movement therapy (CIMT) for the weak arm of a patient attending an outpatient stroke rehabilitation program, the ambulatory care nurse expects to:

a. Constrain the uninvolved arm.
b. Constrain the involved arm.
c. Force use of the weakened arm 50% of the day.
d. Avoid forced use of the weakened arm.

104. An athlete runner was wearing new shoes that felt too tight. The runner complains of pain in the posterior aspect of the heel, especially when running uphill or on soft ground, and has a persistent limp when walking. These are characteristics of:

a. Achilles tendinitis
b. Ankle strain
c. Ankle sprain
d. Achilles bursitis

105. Who bears the ultimate risk of liability when an informed consent is not obtained?

a. The nurse
b. The manager or chief executive officer of a facility or unit
c. The patient
d. The physician

106. A marching band member complains of pain in the bottom of the heel after a long march in a parade and walks with a limp to avoid discomfort. The most likely diagnosis is:

a. Ankle sprain
b. Achilles bursitis
c. Fat pad contusion
d. Plantar warts

107. One of the principles of motivational interviewing is support of self-efficacy, which means that the ambulatory care nurse should:

a. Avoid conflict with the patient when the patient shows resistance to change.
b. Help the patient come to the realization that change is possible.
c. Show appreciation and understanding for the patient's perceptions.
d. Help the patient to recognize the discrepancy between goals and behavior.

108. If a patient has repeatedly missed appointments and failed to follow through with treatments, the best approach when addressing this with the patient is:

a. "How can I help you to manage your healthcare more effectively?"
b. "Your health will not improve until you better manage your treatment."
c. "Why do you miss appointments and fail to follow through with treatments?"
d. "I feel frustrated that I can't seem to convey the importance of your healthcare."

109. The most common type of fracture in postmenopausal women is the:

a. Hip fracture
b. Wrist fracture
c. Vertebral fracture
d. Ankle fracture

110. If a Medicare patient has requested referral for acupuncture to treat chronic pain, the Advance Beneficiary Notice (ABN):

a. Is required because acupuncture is not covered by Medicare
b. Is not required because acupuncture is covered by Medicare
c. May be voluntarily issued to the patient to notify the patient of non-coverage
d. Cannot be issued to the patient because acupuncture is never covered

111. The most important factor in decreasing delay in reimbursement for insurance claims is to:

a. Obtain accurate demographic information about patients.
b. Appeal claims that are denied.
c. Remind patients that they are responsible for unpaid claims.
d. Establish good working relationships with insurance companies.

112. When administering the Mantoux tuberculin skin test, the ambulatory care nurse should advise the patient to return for examination in:

a. 12-24 hours
b. 24-48 hours
c. 48-72 hours
d. 72-96 hours

113. Which of the following does NOT generally require mandatory reporting?

a. Elder abuse
b. Child abuse
c. Intimate partner abuse
d. Vulnerable adult abuse

114. The most critical intervention for a patient with high-altitude cerebral edema is:

a. Oxygen administration
b. Acetazolamide
c. Dexamethasone
d. Descent to a lower elevation

115. In staffing, *locum tenens* refers to:

a. Healthcare providers who work only on an on-call basis
b. Healthcare providers who can decide whether or not to work open shifts
c. Temporarily employed healthcare providers, contracted to provide services for a specified period of time
d. Temporarily employed healthcare providers who work only during certain seasons when populations in an area increase

116. A common medication used for treatment of primary polycythemia is:

a. Hydroxyurea
b. Corticosteroids
c. Erythropoietin
d. Gentamicin

117. If a patient's hemoglobin is 14.0 g/dL, the ambulatory care nurse expects that the hematocrit will be approximately:

a. 28%
b. 36%
c. 42%
d. 48%

118. An adult patient's white blood count (WBC) and differential show:

- WBC: 14,000
- Bands: 11%
- Neutrophils: 72%
- Lymphocytes: 23%
- Monocytes: 2%
- Eosinophils: 2%
- Basophils: 1%

These values are suggestive of:

a. Normal findings
b. Bacterial infection
c. Viral infection
d. Fungal infection

119. When educating staff on the use of new technology, the type of instruction that involves moving around the classroom and monitoring progress rather than lecturing is:

a. Just-in-time presentation
b. One-on-one instruction
c. Group instruction
d. Over-the-shoulder instruction

120. When doing point-of-care testing for the INR, such as with the CoaguChek XS Professional Meter, the blood sample must be placed on the test strip within:

a. 5 seconds of obtaining the sample
b. 15 seconds of obtaining the sample
c. 30 seconds of obtaining the sample
d. 45 seconds of obtaining the sample

121. Episodic care is characterized by being:

a. One-time or limited
b. Part of an ongoing professional relationship
c. Integral to primary care
d. Central to the care of chronic illness

122. Violent and aggressive behavior is most likely to occur with long-term abuse of:

a. Marijuana
b. Cocaine
c. Crack cocaine
d. LSD

123. According to Bloom's original taxonomy of learning (1956), which of the following learning objectives has the highest level of complexity?

a. Comprehension
b. Analysis
c. Application
d. Evaluation

124. If a coworker documents administration of taken-as-needed opioid medications much more frequently than other nursing staff and reports wasting excessive amounts of drugs, the ambulatory care nurse should suspect:

a. Diversion
b. Carelessness
c. Empathy with patients
d. Negligence

125. The primary purpose of a preanesthetic medical examination is:

a. To inform the patient about anesthesia
b. To satisfy a checklist
c. To conduct a risk assessment
d. To answer patient questions about the procedure

126. A patient has difficulty concentrating and focusing attention, has a narrow perceptual field that includes only the immediate task, and has episodes of dry mouth, gastrointestinal (GI) upset, diaphoresis, and palpitations. The patient's level of anxiety would be classified as:

a. Mild
b. Moderate
c. Severe
d. Panic

127. Which of the following is a maladaptive response to stress and anxiety?

a. Setting expectations
b. Mental imagery
c. Self-talk
d. Procrastination

128. In an outpatient surgery center, which of the following is a role that is primarily the responsibility of the circulating nurse?

a. Preparing instruments and equipment
b. Participating in the procedural pause
c. Handing instruments to the surgeon
d. Coordinating care

129. The nurse washes her hands or uses hand sanitizer when coming into the patient room and uses gloves when doing a procedure. What purpose do these procedures demonstrate?

a. Droplet precautions
b. Standard precautions
c. Individual preference for patient-care practices
d. Contact precautions

130. When assisting a patient with smoking cessation, the first step that the ambulatory care nurse should advise the patient to do is to:

a. Throw away all cigarettes and smoking supplies.
b. Tell all family and friends of the plan to quit.
c. Avoid situations that trigger smoking.
d. Set a quit date.

131. The four characteristics that define hazardous waste materials are:

a. Harmful, toxic, active, and reactive
b. Ignitable, corrosive, reactive, and toxic
c. Harmful, ignitable, explosive, and corrosive
d. Harmful, explosive, toxic, and ignitable

132. Which information on a sign-in sheet is a violation of the Health Insurance Portability and Accountability Act of 1996 (HIPAA) Privacy Rule?

a. Name: J. S. Smith
b. Appointment time: 9:30 AM
c. Reason for visit: blood pressure check
d. Appointment with: Dr. Jones

133. A primary difference between obstructive sleep apnea and central sleep apnea is that:

a. With central sleep apnea, no inspiratory effort occurs during apneic periods.
b. With central sleep apnea, there is inspiratory effort during apneic periods.
c. With obstructive sleep apnea, no inspiratory effort occurs during apneic periods.
d. With obstructive sleep apnea, a Cheyne-Stokes breathing pattern occurs.

134. If a physician in a clinic was delayed, resulting in three patients having to reschedule appointments after waiting for extended periods, the first step necessary for service recovery is to:

a. Explain the reason for the delay.
b. Note that patients should expect delays.
c. Apologize.
d. Act as though there is no problem.

135. An 86-year-old patient with Alzheimer's disease is accompanied to a physician's office by her daughter, who is also the patient's caregiver. The daughter states, "I don't understand why she is so stubborn! She's perfectly capable of dressing herself!" This statement is probably an indication of:

a. Elder abuse
b. Caregiver stress
c. Poor family dynamics
d. Low health literacy

136. If a patient has rheumatoid arthritis and is able to carry out usual activities, such as self-care and work, but is limited in carrying out other activities, such as sports and household chores, the patient's functional status is:

a. Class 4
b. Class 3
c. Class 2
d. Class 1

137. One of the primary advantages of an urgent care center over a hospital emergency department is:

a. The staff members are usually better trained.
b. The cost is generally lower.
c. The access is usually more convenient.
d. The equipment is usually more up to date.

138. If a patient with diabetes takes insulin, this type of therapy is classified as:

a. Replacement
b. Prophylactic
c. Acute
d. Palliative

139. A patient complains of postmastectomy breast pain syndrome. This is an example of which type of neuropathic pain?

a. Central
b. Peripheral
c. Sympathetically maintained
d. Differentiation

140. If a patient received staples for a laceration on an arm, the patient should be advised to return for staple removal within:

a. 3-5 days
b. 5-7 days
c. 7-10 days
d. 10-14 days

141. Which of the following is NOT covered by workers' compensation insurance?

a. Injury during the commute to or from work
b. Injury at a mandatory-attendance company-sponsored sports activity
c. Injury during travel for company-sponsored business
d. Injury in the company parking lot while walking into the building

142. If a patient has a subungual (beneath the nail) hematoma and is to have it drained by a cautery needle, the first step is to:

a. Drape the digit with sterile 4×4-inch gauze pads.
b. Soak the digit in warm povidone-iodine or antiseptic soap solution for 5 minutes.
c. Provide the patient with an analgesic.
d. Activate the cautery needle so it has time to heat.

143. If an older female patient with moderately advanced dementia is cradling a doll and says, "This is my baby," and refuses to relinquish the doll for an examination, which of the following is the most appropriate response?

a. "That is a doll and not a baby."
b. "I'll hold the baby for you."
c. "I won't bother your baby."
d. "You must give me the doll."

144. A patient who has come to an ambulatory care center many times is disabled and wheelchair-bound, and lifting the patient onto the table for examination is very difficult. The best solution is probably to:

a. Ask the patient to bring along someone to help lift.
b. Examine the patient in the wheelchair.
c. Ensure that one examining table is wheelchair accessible.
d. Advise the patient to seek medical care elsewhere.

145. The ambulatory care nurse has called a patient who is being treated for chronic depression because the patient has missed one appointment and two sessions of the support group. Which of the following statements by the patient would be the most concerning?

a. "I don't like the support team leader, so I don't feel comfortable."
b. "I've been giving all my things away, and I feel so much better."
c. "I know that I need to keep my appointments, and I'll do better."
d. "My partner will be upset with me for not going to therapy."

146. In a just culture, if an ambulatory care nurse misreads a medication order and administers an incorrect dosage of a medication, the response should be to:

a. Take punitive action.
b. Coach the nurse.
c. Place the nurse on probation.
d. Review procedures and console the nurse.

147. Following fine-needle aspiration of a breast lesion, patient instructions should include:

a. No special care is necessary.
b. Apply a pressure dressing and ice packs for 24 hours.
c. Alternate warm and cold compresses for 24-48 hours.
d. Take an opioid to relieve discomfort as needed.

148. In ambulatory care, the individual most in control of patient care is the:

a. Patient
b. Physician
c. Nurse
d. Family

149. A patient with a history of Addison's disease (primary adrenal insufficiency) comes to the emergency department with hypotension and loss of consciousness, which was preceded by nausea, vomiting, abdominal pain, and confusion. Immediate intervention should be:

a. Laboratory tests (complete blood count, electrolytes, cortisol level, and thyroid function)
b. Hydrocortisone 100 mg IV over 30 seconds
c. 1,000 mL of 5% dextrose in 0.9% saline
d. Abdominal computed tomography

150. In leadership, span of control refers to:

a. The number of patients served in a unit
b. The number of individuals a leader supervises
c. The number of departments a leader supervises
d. The decision-making authority of a leader

Answer Key and Explanations for Test #2

1. A: Conflict resolution should begin by asking each participant to state his or her position without interruption. In reaching a solution, collaboration and cooperation are usually more effective than coercion.

2. B: If a patient with a history of atrial fibrillation takes warfarin as an anticoagulant, the patient's INR should usually remain between 2 and 3, with a value greater than 4.9 being considered a critical value. If the INR is elevated (<5) without evidence of bleeding, omitting a dose of warfarin may be effective; if the INR is excessively elevated (>5 to <9) without bleeding, up to two doses should be withheld. If severe bleeding occurs, then fresh frozen plasma with 10 mg of vitamin K may be administered.

3. C: The temperature in operating rooms is usually maintained at 68 °F (20 °C) to 73 °F (23 °C) to help prevent hypothermia while maintaining the comfort level for staff. The decontamination area is maintained cooler, at 60 °F (16 °C) to 65 °F (18 °C), to discourage the growth of microorganisms. Temperatures in the post-anesthesia care unit and cardiac catheterization lab are higher at 70 °F (21 °C) to 76 °F (24 °C).

Humidity should be maintained between 20% and 60%. Humidity of 50% to 60% reduces the production of static electricity associated with electrosurgery.

4. D: The Food and Drug Administration's roles include:

- Regulating medical devices, such as respirators, to ensure that they are safe to use and that safety hazards are identified.
- Inspecting manufacturing facilities and conducting sampling and tests to ensure workers and the public are protected from electronic product radiation.
- Ensuring that state standards meet minimum federal requirements.
- Ensuring the safety of drugs, vaccines, and biological products.
- Protecting employees who report violations of food/drug handling/production or refuse to participate in work-required violations.

5. A: Ambulatory care nurses may be liable for improper administration of drugs, failing to follow standard medical procedures, failure to follow a physician's orders or take correct oral or verbal orders, failure to report changes in patients' conditions or defective equipment, miscounting sponges/instruments/surgical equipment, avoidable injuries to patients from falls or burns, and mishandling of patients' personal belongings.

6. B: Handheld core biopsy devices typically use a 14-gauge needle. The sample is large enough that it can be tested for biological markers. The outpatient procedure is done under local anesthetic and often with ultrasound image guidance to avoid sampling errors associated with improper positioning of the needle.

7. D: Personal health information that is protected includes:

- Any information about an individual's past, present, or future health or condition (mental or physical)
- Provision of healthcare provided to the individual

- Any information related to payment for healthcare services that can be used to identify the person
- Identifying information (name, address, Social Security number, birthdate) and any document or material that contains the identifying information (such as laboratory records)

8. C: Combined hormonal contraceptives contain a synthetic form of estrogen, most often ethinyl estradiol, and a progestin, which has a progesterone-like action. Estradiol prevents the development of a dominant follicle, and the progestin prevents the luteinizing hormone surge, so ovulation does not occur. With perfect use, the failure rate of oral combined contraceptives is about 0.3%, but with average use (which includes occasionally forgetting), the failure rate is 8%, so patients must understand the importance of consistent use.

9. B: Vesicular breath sounds are the normal breath sounds expected to be heard on auscultation of the peripheral lung fields. They are soft and low-pitched and indicate healthy lungs. Ronchi are low-pitched sounds similar to snoring that occur when air is passing through mucus or a partially blocked airway, as in pneumonia. Rales are soft rattling sounds on inhalation that can further be described as coarse, fine, dry, or moist. Rales are also heard with pneumonia. Wheezes are high-pitched sounds on inhalation or exhalation, sometimes audible without a stethoscope, indicating narrowing airways, such as in an asthma exacerbation.

10. B: Categories of HIPAA violations and the associated penalties:

Category	Description	Penalties
1	A violation that the entity was not aware of and could not avoid if exercising reasonable effort to follow HIPAA rules.	Fines of $100 to $50,000 per violation up to a maximum of $1.5 million.
2	A violation that the entity should have recognized but could not avoid even if exercising reasonable effort.	Fines of $100 to $50,000 per violation up to a maximum of $1.5 million.
3	A violation resulting from "willful neglect" of HIPAA rules, but the entity tried to correct the violation.	Fines of $10,000 to $50,000 per violation up to a maximum of $1.5 million.
4	A violation resulting from "willful neglect" of HIPAA rules, and the entity made no effort to correct the violation.	Fines of $50,000 to a maximum of $1.5 million per violation.

11. C: This finding is commonly found with pyelonephritis (or interstitial nephritis) because it indicates an infective or inflammatory process. Hyaline casts are found with concentrated urine, such as in those who are febrile or are taking diuretics. Red cell casts occur with glomerulonephritis. Renal tubular cell casts are found with acute tubular necrosis and interstitial nephritis. Broad, waxy casts are common to chronic kidney disease, and coarse granular casts are nonspecific but can be found with interstitial nephritis.

12. D: Lithium is a simple salt, so the intake of sodium in the diet can affect lithium levels. Decreased intake may cause lithium levels to increase, and increased intake may cause them to decrease. Patients should be advised to have a consistent intake of sodium in their diets. Caffeine has a similar effect on lithium. Lithium can react with numerous drugs as well.

13. C: Medication errors cause injury to up to 1.5 million people each year and result in thousands of deaths; therefore, reducing medication errors should be a priority for all healthcare providers. Studies show that drugs commonly involved in incident reports include chemotherapeutic agents, anticoagulants, opiates, and opioids. Most errors occur during the dispensing of drugs, followed by errors in prescribing or ordering drugs. Incidents include delays in administration of drugs, incorrect dose, incorrect patient, and failing to administer a dose.

14. A: Patient teaching should include the importance of drinking extra fluids to prevent the formation of kidney stones and urinary crystals. Patients should also be advised to use a sunscreen and avoid exposure to direct sunlight because sulfasalazine can cause increased sensitivity to the sun. Some patients may experience an orange-yellow discoloration of the urine. Sulfasalazine should be stored at room temperature and should be protected from excessive heat or moisture.

15. D: The following table lists several educational models and how they are implemented.

Model	Description
Goal focused	Learners are presented with a goal, and all materials and activities are aimed at achieving that goal.
Guided focus	Learning takes place outside of the formal classroom with materials provided or recommended by the instructor.
Anchored	Activities are based on problem solving in relation to realistic case studies.
Collaborative	Learners work together to complete a learning activity or project.
Project based	Learners develop materials (videos, web pages, pamphlets) regarding a topic.
Problem based	Learners work in teams to solve problems.
Direct instruction	Instructor-focused presentation.

16. B: Both urine dipstick and blood glucose are the most appropriate for a teenager with fruity breath and sleepiness, and would provide the fastest results to allow for rapid treatment in the case of diabetic ketoacidosis, which is considered a medical emergency. The urine dipstick may show whether ketones are in the urine, which indicates diabetic ketoacidosis when in conjunction with a severely high blood glucose level. The clinician can then use this information to determine if diabetes is suspected or if another avenue of diagnosis should be pursued. Positive ketones and high blood glucose levels would indicate that the teen should be further evaluated for diabetes. HbA1c will be a good diagnostic tool for diabetes, but takes more time to result, and therefore should be taken after a definitive diagnosis is determined.

17. B: A patient who is diagnosed with Huntington's disease (an autosomal-dominant disorder) has a 50% chance of passing on the disorder to each child because the child only needs to inherit the defective gene from one parent. There is no treatment that will alter the course of the disease, although some medications may help to ease symptoms. Because there is no treatment, testing of children is not advised unless they show signs of juvenile onset (rare).

18. A: Kolb's learning styles inventory outlines a preferred style of learning as follows:

- **Accommodative**: Prefers to learn through a combination of concrete experience and active experimentation, solves problems through trial and error, and tends to complete tasks.
- **Assimilative**: Prefers abstract concepts and reflective observation and is more interested in abstract ideas than people and applying ideas.

- **Divergent**: Prefers concrete experience and reflective observations, is imaginative with good ideas, and is emotional. Likes working with people.
- **Convergent**: Prefers abstract concepts and active experimentation and prefers dealing with things to people.

19. D: A respiratory nebulizer treatment would be the first treatment of choice to assist this patient with wheezing and shortness of breath. Steroids may be indicated, but are not the initial treatment in this setting, and may be considered after a nebulizer treatment fails to relieve the systems. A urine dipstick and blood glucose monitoring are not immediately needed with a complaint of wheezing.

20. C: Bell's palsy may appear similar to a stroke, but a stroke does not cause hyperacusis or an impaired sense of taste. About 60% of cases resolve without any treatment, although most are treated with prednisone because this makes complete recovery more likely.

21. B: The critical elements of a disaster plan include:

- **Communication plans**: Phone trees or other notification systems, and plans for external notification of community agencies/resources, should be established.
- **Essential supplies**: IVs, dressing supplies, and essential medications should be stockpiled.
- **Staff roles and responsibilities**: Staff members are trained in disaster preparedness and understand their roles and responsibilities.
- **Power/utilities**: Backup systems should provide power for up to 96 hours.
- **Clinical patient care**: Plans for provision of care under varying circumstances, including alternate plans, should be established.

22. C: Normal values should be 1,800–2,000. A significant risk exists when the ANC falls to 1,000, and the risk is severe and life-threatening at 500. The ANC decreases when not enough neutrophils are produced or too many are destroyed. Neutropenia is usually diagnosed with blood tests because symptoms are nonspecific until the patient develops an infection.

23. D: The three stages of chemotherapy for leukemia are:

- **Induction**: Chemotherapy agents wipe out leukemic cells, and normal myeloid cells as well, over a 4- to 6-week period, resulting in neutropenia and thrombocytopenia.
- **Consolidation**: Treatment continues for 4–8 months at lower dosages to kill any remaining cancerous cells.
- **Maintenance**: Some type of treatment may continue for up to 3 years while the patient is monitored closely.

24. C: According to the Institute for Healthcare Improvement, patient safety rounds should be conducted at least every week, usually by multidisciplinary teams. Doing so on a regularly scheduled basis helps the staff appreciate the organization's commitment to safety. The safety rounds should be carried out in every department involved in patient care. They should involve not only observing staff, patients, and equipment in the environment, but also questioning and taking time to listen to staff members and taking opportunities to teach about safety.

25. A: The lifetime risk of developing breast cancer with these mutations is 50% to 85%. Whereas the average female has a 2% lifetime risk of developing ovarian cancer, those with the BRCA1 mutation have up to a 46% risk; those with the BRCA2 mutation have up to a 27% risk. Many women with these mutations choose to undergo elective mastectomies and oophorectomies.

26. D: RCA is a retrospective attempt to determine the cause of an adverse event. RCA involves interviews, observations, and review of medical records. Often, an extensive questionnaire is completed by the professional doing the RCA, essentially tracing every step in the patient's hospitalization and care, including every treatment, every medication, and every contact. The focus of the RCA is on systems and processes rather than on individuals. In many cases, an adverse event is the result of a series of errors or a system of problems rather than one clearly identifiable process failure.

27. C: When irrigating a wound with normal saline, the irrigation pressure should be 10–15 psi, as a pressure greater than 15 psi may cause trauma. A pressure lower than 4 psi cannot adequately cleanse a wound of debris. A bulb syringe, for example, usually delivers less than 2 psi of pressure. A pressure of 8 psi can be achieved with a 35 mL syringe and a 19-gauge needle. A wound irrigation device allows more accurate pressure control, and many come with a shield to prevent splashing.

28. B: The purpose of sterilization and disinfection is to prevent disease transmission from patient to patient, or patient to staff. Sterilization is the destruction of all microorganisms on a surface through both chemical and physical means, while disinfection eliminates most pathogens (except spores) using chemicals. Sterilization and disinfection are regulated by the EPA and FDA with guidelines supported by the CDC.

29. A: All members of the staff should be encouraged to participate in process evaluation and improvement. Formal processes for improvement can be carried out, especially in larger organizations; but simply identifying one process that needs improvement, and working to find solutions to improve that process, can be the start of process improvement in any organization.

30. B: A first-degree burn is superficial and affects only the epidermis, such as occurs with sunburn. A second-degree burn often has sloughing of the dermis; large blisters; red, weeping, exposed tissue; and considerable pain. Third-degree burns are more serious and extend through the dermis and into the tissues underlying the dermis, such as the vessels, nerves, and muscles. Because the nerves may be damaged, there is less pain associated with third-degree burns than second-degree burns.

31. C: Advocacy is working for the best interests of the patient despite personal values in conflict and assisting patients to have access to appropriate resources. Although parents are usually barred from surgical areas, it may be in the best interest of the child to make an exception for a child that is particularly anxious.

32. A: The following table contains descriptions of the stages of irradiation damage.

Stage I	Slight edema and inflammation. Dilation and increased permeability of capillaries result in erythema, itching, burning, or pain.
Stage II	The skin is dry, itching, and scaly with partial sloughing of the epidermis.
Stage III	The skin is moist and blistering with a loss of epidermal tissue, serous drainage, and increased pain.
Stage IV	Permanent hair loss, tissue atrophy, changes in pigment, and ulcerations.

33. B: An example of therapeutic communication is "I see that you are upset" because this is an empathetic observation. The ambulatory care nurse should avoid directly asking for explanations of behavior (e.g., "Oh, my goodness, why are you so upset?") that do not directly affect care. The nurse should also avoid meaningless clichés (e.g., "Don't worry, I'm sure everything will be all right") and advice (e.g., "You should consider further treatments").

34. A: With urine dipstick testing, a positive result for nitrites or leukocyte esterase is likely an indication of urinary tract infection because these are products of white blood cells, which increase with infection. A positive result for bilirubin may indicate a liver disorder. A positive result for ketones may be a sign of diabetes. Protein is often found in the urine in small amounts, but if the amount is significant, this could be a sign of renal disease.

35. C: In a leadership role, an effective strategy for giving feedback about an issue to another nurse includes:

- Being objective and specific about the issue.
- Avoiding judgmental statements.
- Providing positive and negative feedback rather than focusing only on negative feedback.
- Giving feedback immediately, whether positive or negative.
- Providing frequent constructive feedback.
- Giving negative feedback only in private and maintaining confidentiality.
- Providing feedback based on observed behavior, with specific descriptions rather than generalities.
- Encouraging the individual to also give feedback and express feelings.
- Providing suggestions for change or methods to use to find a solution to a problem.

36. B: If a person has been drinking alcohol, it is absorbed into the bloodstream within about 30 minutes and is metabolized at the rate of about one-quarter ounce per hour. Thus, if a person is drinking heavily, the blood alcohol level can increase much faster than the body can metabolize the alcohol, increasing the risk of alcohol poisoning. Following the last drink that a person has, the blood alcohol level will continue to increase for the next 30-40 minutes.

37. A: Approaches to conflict resolution include:

Accommodating	One party ceding to the other, usually when the other has more power.
Avoiding	Taking steps to avoid dealing with the conflict.
Collaborating	Trying to find a solution that pleases both parties.
Competing	One party trying to win at all costs.
Compromising	Each party ceding something in return for harmony.
Confronting	Using "I" messages and assertive problem solving.
Forcing	One party issuing orders to force a solution.
Negotiating	Similar to collaborating, with back-and-forth bargaining.
Reassuring	Attempting to make everyone happy.
Problem solving	Trying to find a solution that works for everyone using a step-by-step approach
Withdrawing	One party withdrawing from the conflict, leaving the conflict unresolved.

38. D: Cocaine increases levels of dopamine by binding to the dopamine receptors so that dopamine is not removed at the synapse. As dopamine levels increase, this reinforces the reward system of the brain so the person needs higher doses to achieve the same effects. Cocaine acts quickly, in about 15-30 minutes for those snorting cocaine and 5-10 minutes for those injecting or smoking it, but the sensations are short lived, so users often take repeat hits.

39. B: POS Codes comprise two digits. Commonly used POS Codes include:

01	Pharmacy	**19**	Off-campus hospital outpatient
02	Telehealth	**20**	Urgent care facility
11	Office	**22**	On-campus hospital outpatient
15	Mobile unit	**23**	Emergency room, hospital
17	Walk-in retail clinic	**24**	Ambulatory surgical center
18	Worksite	**49**	Independent clinic

40. D: Screening is recommended for all women 65 and older, as well as women 60-64 with increased risk factors. The Bone Health and Osteoporosis Foundation extends the recommendations to include all men 70 and older as well as those at risk. Osteoporosis is diagnosed with a DEXA score of –2.5 or lower in the spine, femoral neck, or total hip. Osteopenia is diagnosed with a score between –2.5 and –1.5. A normal value is –0.1 or higher.

41. B: Critical pathways give specific interventions and measurable outcomes for the healthcare team, allowing them to evaluate each patient with a certain list of symptoms and expected results against unexpected or bad results. Payroll doesn't directly relate to performance improvement, but the payroll department would have their own set of performance criteria. Tracer methodology is used to identify hazards in the work process, geared toward patient safety rather than performance improvement overall. A cost-benefit analysis presents the overall benefits of a new intervention by balancing those benefits against the costs as a method of arguing for approval of the new intervention.

42. A: The first-line drug of choice for treatment of type 2 diabetes mellitus is metformin. It is relatively inexpensive, has been used for many years, and is well tolerated by most patients. If the metformin is not able to lower the serum glucose level, then another drug, such as a sulfonylurea, is often added to the metformin. Some newer drugs that are on the market have cardiovascular and renal benefits as well as controlling glucose levels, but they are costly, and some have serious adverse effects.

43. D: Other examples of nonbillable services include dental care and routine foot care (such as nail trimming). Medicare does not cover long-term custodial care, routine eye examination and eyeglasses, chiropractic services, and cosmetic surgeries. Most immunizations are covered by Medicare Part D, but the COVID-19, hepatitis B, flu, and pneumococcal vaccines are covered by Medicare Part B. If a patient may have been exposed to a microorganism, Medicare Part B will also reimburse for tetanus or rabies vaccinations.

44. C: If a patient has developed herpes zoster (shingles), treatment with antivirals should begin within 72 hours and should continue for 1 week. The drugs of choice are valacyclovir or famciclovir. These medications reduce the duration of the lesions and episodes of pain but do not prevent postherpetic syndrome. Corticosteroids are also sometimes given to speed healing. The vaccine to prevent herpes zoster is recommended for all healthy adults older than age 50.

45. B: Approximately 80% to 90% of modifiable contributors to healthy outcomes is attributed to social determinants of health with the remaining 10% to 20% attributed to medical treatment. One of the leading indicators of health is the person's place of residence because this relates to security in housing, food, income, education, and access to healthcare. Place of residence is also directly linked to life expectancy. Sometimes the difference of a few miles into a different zip code can mean a difference in years of life expectancy.

46. D: The recommended treatment for chlamydial infection (*C. trachomatis)* for adolescents and adults is doxycycline 100 mg orally BID for 7 days. Chlamydial infections are the most common bacterial infections in the US, especially among those age 24 and younger. Treatments for other sexually transmitted infections include:

- Syphilis: Benzathine penicillin G, 2.4 million units IM.
- Gonorrhea: Ceftriaxone 500 mg IM.
- Trichomoniasis: Metronidazole 500 mg BID for 7 days.

47. C: Millions of children's diets are insufficient for adequate growth and development. Additionally, with food insecurity, the food that is often most readily available is usually high in fats and simple carbohydrates, leading to obesity and associated illnesses such as hypertension and diabetes. Programs such as the Special Supplemental Nutrition Program for Women, Infants, and Children (commonly known as the WIC program), the Supplemental Nutrition Assistance Program (SNAP), and free school lunches are critically important for this population.

48. A: Sinusitis is caused by the common cold virus and usually resolves without treatment within 7-10 days, but if it persists, there may be a bacterial infection that requires antibiotics. Warm, moist compresses may help to relieve any discomfort.

49. D: Bleeding gums may indicate myelosuppression, which can result in thrombocytopenia, agranulocytosis, and leukopenia. The thrombocytopenia particularly increases the risk of bleeding. Fatigue, general malaise, nausea, and diarrhea are very common adverse effects. Patients usually receive an emetic before and after treatment to relieve nausea and vomiting.

50. A: Many prisoners are substance abusers before their incarceration, and drugs are widely available within prison populations despite efforts to limit access. Drugs are also often available in transitional housing that is available to offenders after discharge. The National Institute on Drug Abuse estimates that 85% of the prison population has a substance use disorder, with marijuana and cocaine or crack being the most commonly used drugs.

51. B: If the patient is taking insulin glargine (which typically works over the course of 24 hours) once daily in the evening and is to add rapid-acting insulin lispro before each meal, the patient should eat the meals within 15 minutes to avoid an insulin reaction. Alternatively, the patient could take the insulin lispro immediately after finishing the meal. Insulin lispro is a genetically modified form of insulin.

52. A: Sign language interpreters should be used for important communication (face the patient, not the interpreter) because lip reading is not 100% accurate. Assistive devices, such as writing materials, TDD, and phone/relay service, should be available for use. Do not chew, smoke, or eat while speaking to the patient.

53. D: The nurse should pull the pinna up and back to straighten the ear canal so that the irrigation is more effective. If the irrigation is for a child younger than age 6, the pinna should be pulled down and back. Ear irrigation is typically done to remove impacted cerumen that occludes the tympanic membrane or to remove foreign objects. A syringe or a Waterpik can be used to flush the ear.

54. B: Patients with global aphasia have difficulty understanding and producing language in speaking, reading, and writing, although patients may understand gestures. Some trial and error may be necessary to determine the best means of communication.

55. A: The nurse expects that the patient will exhibit purposeful response to verbal/tactile stimuli (this does not include a reflex response to pain). Spontaneous ventilation should be adequate without the need for an airway intervention. Cardiovascular function is usually maintained without intervention. The patient must be monitored continuously, with medicines and equipment readily available for rescue from oversedation.

56. A: Microsocial advocacy is aimed at the individual patient and the patient's family. This is the form of advocacy that is most generally practiced by ambulatory care nurses. However, advocacy at the macrosocial level is equally important. Macrosocial advocacy is aimed at service organizations, community populations, and global (national and international) populations. Macrosocial advocacy includes participation in the development and implementation of policies in order to influence public policy.

57. A: Blood flow through a vascular access for dialysis should be maintained at greater than or equal to 300 mL per minute, with prescriptions ranging from 300-600 mL/min. If the flow slows to less than 300 mL/min, this indicates dysfunction of the access, and there is an increased risk of thrombus formation. Low graft blood flow may indicate stenosis of the graft or the venous outflow. Other causes of low graft blood flow include low arterial inflow (associated with atherosclerosis or fibromuscular hyperplasia), hypotension, and technical error in administration.

58. C: If treatments must begin immediately, then the patient should carry out the procedure while lying supine to help control leakage, with a low exchange volume and shorter-than-usual dwell period, especially with the initial treatments. Patients may choose a continuous or intermittent process and manual or automated.

59. B: Although a number of accrediting and certification agencies are active, the Joint Commission is an accrediting and a certifying agency for healthcare organizations, including those involved in ambulatory care. Accreditation requires extensive preparation and compliance with health and safety standards. Certification requires compliance with standards and engagement in improvement activities.

60. A: According to SAMHSA, the three E's of trauma are:

- Events: These include the traumatic event that occurred once or repeatedly and that may be physically or psychologically harmful.
- Experiences: These are the personal perception and experience of the traumatic event. Individuals may experience a traumatic event very differently, with some perceiving an event as traumatic and others not.
- Effects: These are the long-acting adverse effects experienced by the person because of the traumatic event.

61. D: Medicare C refers to Medicare Advantage plans, which are essentially plans that combine Medicare Part A (hospital benefits), Medicare Part B (medical benefits), and sometimes Medicare Part D (prescription drug benefits). This form of Medicare is offered by private insurance companies contract with CMS. Such companies typically provide a benefits plan that may differ from original Medicare (which includes Parts A and B). Medicare Advantage plans often offer additional benefits, such as vision, dental, and hearing coverage, that are not usually provided by Medicare, but patients are usually restricted to healthcare providers in the plan's network.

62. C: This clear nasal discharge may represent a leakage of cerebrospinal fluid from torn meninges resulting from fracture of the cribriform plate. A drop of clear drainage should be placed on filter paper and examined for a clear area around a central stain of blood. If cerebrospinal fluid drainage is suspected, the patient should be placed upright, have a CT scan, and have a neurological consult.

63. A: Smartphones are ubiquitous, and many adults rely almost exclusively on text messaging for communication. HIPAA-compliant text messaging software is available. Some types of messaging (such as accounting and billing information and collection notices) require written consent to send. Some other types of messages (such as appointment reminders, laboratory results, medical instructions, and notices of prescriptions) do not require consent. However, it is good practice to ask for consent before sending any type of message.

64. B: Only permanent teeth are reimplanted, not primary teeth. The procedure is as follows:

- Cleanse the tooth with sterile normal saline or Hanks' solution, avoiding any disruption of the fibers.
- If the tooth has been dry for 20–60 minutes, soak the tooth in Hanks' solution for 30 minutes.
- If the tooth has been dry for >60 minutes, soak the tooth in citric acid for 5 minutes, 2% stannous fluoride for 5 minutes, and doxycycline solution for 5 minutes.
- Remove the clot in the socket and gently irrigate the socket with normal saline.
- Place the tooth firmly into the socket, cover it with gauze, and have the patient bite firmly on the gauze until splinting is applied.
- Apply splinting material and mold packing over the implanted tooth and two adjacent teeth on both sides (encompassing five teeth).

65. A: The Payne-Martin Classification System for Skin Tears categories include:

- Category I: Skin tear leaves avulsed skin adequate to cover the wound. Tears may be full-thickness linear or partial-thickness flap-type.
- Category II: Skin tear with loss of partial thickness, involving scant loss (<25% of epidermal flap over the tear is lost) to moderate-large loss (>25% of dermis in the tear is lost).
- Category III: Skin tear with complete loss of tissue, involving a partial-thickness wound with no epidermal flap.

66. C: Patient engagement develops along a continuum that ranges from very little to maximal input:

- Lowest: Patient receives direct treatment with consent
- Next level: Patient receives information about his or her diagnosis
- Next level: Patient is asked about preferences when developing a treatment plan
- Highest level: Patient's preferences and best practices guide treatment

The patient should be an active participant in all decisions regarding care and should be provided adequate education so that the patient can make informed decisions.

67. D: The patient is at risk for Lyme disease, which is spread through a tick bite. These signs and symptoms are consistent with early-stage infection, but Lyme disease can cause severe infection resulting in Lyme arthritis, neurologic Lyme, and Lyme carditis. Treatment includes oral antibiotics (such as doxycycline, amoxicillin, or cefuroxime axetil), usually for 2-3 weeks.

68. B: This is a common indication of low health literacy. Other indications include paperwork that is not filled out properly, missing appointments, failing to adhere to a medication/treatment plan, and absence of follow-through for referrals for laboratory tests or specialist care.

69. D: The CD4 count that indicates a change in diagnosis to AIDS is less than 200 cell/mm^3. The normal CD4 count range is 500-1,600 cell/mm^3. Currently, patients positive for HIV are immediately started on antiretroviral drugs, and the CD4 count is used to monitor progress, usually every 3-6 months. CD4 is a kind of protein that is found on some T lymphocyte cells. The viral load (the number of HIV particles in a milliliter of blood) is also monitored. The viral load should be less than 40-75.

70. D: The nurse should adjust the settings slowly until the patient experiences relief, starting with low settings. TENS devices use two to four electrodes, usually with placement above and below the site of the pain. Controls include the on/off button, the mode (constant, intermittent, bursts, modulation), and the timing.

71. D: Shared decision-making encompasses three steps:

- Choice talk: The healthcare provider provides an overview of options for treatment.
- Option talk: The healthcare provider provides a detailed explanation of options for treatment.
- Decision talk: The patient and healthcare provider make decisions based on patient preferences and input.

In some cases, options for treatment are very limited. But in many cases, several different treatment options may be available, and patients should have an active part in decision-making.

72. C: Perspiration cools the body through evaporation. However, evaporation slows when heat is high and humidity is greater than 75%. With radiation, the heat radiates through the skin. With convection, heat transfers to air moving across the body. Conduction involves the loss of heat into the surrounding air, solids, or liquids. Conduction, convection, and radiation are not effective if the ambient temperature is higher than the body temperature, and they can result in increased body temperature.

73. A: The most effective strategy is to study medical Spanish so that the nurse can speak directly with patients and establish closer relationships. Although having materials printed in Spanish is helpful, some immigrants are not literate in Spanish. An interpreter/translator should always be available (in person or by telephone) for complex cases. Providing information about English classes is not likely to have a significant impact on communication.

74. B: Bats are common carriers of rabies, so any direct contact, especially with a break in the skin, should be treated as though it is positive for rabies. A four-step regimen is available for those who are immunocompetent; a five-step regimen is available for those who are immunocompromised. For those who were previously vaccinated, a two-step postexposure regimen is also available.

75. C: An actinic keratosis is a precancerous lesion. It typically appears as a small scaly or crusty lesion in sun-exposed parts of the body. Acrochordons (skin tags) are benign but are common in those with type 2 diabetes mellitus. Cherry angiomas form from clustered dilated capillaries and are benign; however, if groups of them appear suddenly, this can indicate an underlying malignancy. Seborrheic keratosis is a crusted, wart-like, black-brown raised growth that is unsightly but benign and is most common in older adults.

76. B: Short and simple yes/no questions are easier to comprehend and respond to than questions that ask for evaluation or details. It is important to allow the patient ample time to respond, and to speak to the patient slowly and clearly, maintaining eye contact and offering encouragement.

77. D: The National Institutes of Health recommendations for daily intake of calcium vary according to age and gender:

Age	Male	Female	Pregnant	Lactating
0–6 months	200 mg	200 mg		
7–12 months	260 mg	260 mg		
1–3 years	700 mg	700 mg		
4–8 years	1,000 mg	1,000 mg		
9–13 years	1,300 mg	1,300 mg		
14–18 years	1,300 mg	1,300 mg	1,300 mg	1,300 mg
19–50 years	1,000 mg	1,000 mg	1,000 mg	1,000 mg
51–70 years	1,000 mg	1,200 mg		
>70 years	1,200 mg	1,200 mg		

78. A: The rescue treatment of choice for an acute asthma attack is a SABA, such as albuterol or levalbuterol. SABAs are bronchodilators. The inhaled form is usually used for acute attacks. The next step is a low-dose ICS, such as budesonide or fluticasone. The third step, if the asthma does not improve, is to administer a medium-dose ICS, a LABA, or montelukast. The dosages continue to increase at each step up the treatment ladder.

79. D: These signs are likely indicative of Wernicke-Korsakoff syndrome. The disease is triggered by inadequate diet and thiamine (vitamin B1) deficiency. Wernicke encephalopathy typically occurs first and can be reversed with thiamine treatment. Korsakoff syndrome results in loss of memory, and this cannot be reversed, but thiamine therapy may prevent further damage to the brain.

80. A: The nurse should advise the patient to avoid chewing on the affected side and to avoid any very hot or very cold foods because the extremes of temperature may trigger pain. The patient needs to continue dental care to avoid caries but should use a soft-bristle toothbrush or swab to gently cleanse the right side of the mouth.

81. D: The five A's for developing interventions based on the needs of the individual are:

- **Ask** every individual about their health behaviors.
- **Advise** every individual with unhealthy behaviors to modify that behavior in a manner that is straightforward, strong, and individualized for the person.
- **Assess** the willingness of the individual to change or modify the unhealthy behavior.
- **Assist** the individual to change or modify the behavior.
- **Arrange** for follow-up to ensure the individual has changed or modified the behavior.

82. B: The chronic illnesses most often managed include diabetes mellitus, hypertension, and asthma. The primary roles of the nurse in coordination of care include identifying patients who need coordination of care, carrying out outreach, meeting with patients face to face, providing support for patient engagement, managing cross-setting communication, coaching and counseling, triaging, and participating in group visits.

83. C: Revenue cycle processes include preregistration/registration, provision of billable services, coding, capture (charges documented into billable form), submission, appeals/resubmissions, remittance (receipt of payment and posting), and collection (unpaid bills are referred for collection).

84. A: Symptoms common to other neuromuscular disorders include:

- **Multiple sclerosis**: Tremor, vision impairment, weakness of one or more limbs, and slurred speech.
- **Myasthenia gravis**: Eyelid drooping, diplopia, dysphagia, muscle weakness, and impaired speaking.
- **Muscular dystrophy**: Waddling gait, muscle pain/stiffness, and impaired ability to rise from sitting or lying.

85. D: One of the primary goals in this transition management is the prevention of rehospitalization, so transition management is often an ongoing process rather than a one-time intervention. In this transition, the patient may return to the home but is often still in need of ongoing treatment, such as physical therapy and medication management.

86. B: Although diabetes does not directly cause skin infections, elevated glucose levels lower the ability of the body to fight the infection, and impaired circulation slows healing. Bacterial and fungal infections are common and, in some cases, are the first sign of diabetes.

87. A: The nurse must practice in accordance with the nurse practice act where the care is delivered, not where it originates. The nurse must also be licensed to provide care in both states.

88. C: The five R strategy is:

1. Discuss the **relevance** of making changes to the individual because people like to know up front what is in it for them.
2. Outline all of the **risks** associated with continuing the unhealthy behavior.
3. List and describe the **rewards** associated with changing the behavior.
4. Identify and discuss **roadblocks** to the individual's changing behavior.
5. **Repeat** the five R strategy at each visit with the individual.

89. B: When the nurse is assessing a patient via telehealth, the patient can assist in providing objective information, such as a blood pressure reading of 180/96. Subjective information includes such things as reporting a severe cough, although if the nurse hears or observes the coughing during the telehealth visit, then the information is objective. A complaint of feeling feverish is subjective, but if the patient uses a thermometer to measure the temperature, that finding is objective. Remote monitoring data are also objective.

90. A: Once a nurse agrees to provide services, including accepting patient assignments within a scheduled shift, the nurse has a legal obligation to the patient to ensure continuity of care, and the obligation continues until the patient is transferred to the care of another or is discharged from care.

91. C: DSTs usually provide checklists to make sure that important items are not overlooked. The nurse should always keep in mind that DSTs cannot include all variables; therefore, although they serve as useful guides, they should not supplant independent evaluation and judgment. DSTs should be viewed as support tools only, not as decision-making tools.

92. B: Such accidents must be reported to OSHA within 8 hours, usually by the end of the shift during which the accident occurred. OSHA requires that the workplace be free of hazards, that equipment is safe and properly maintained, and that hazard warning signs be posted. A record must be maintained of all work-related injuries or illnesses, and employees and their representatives should have access to this record.

93. D: The purpose of the eNLC is to provide a multistate license to nurses. Twenty-nine states signed the original eNLC in 2018, and the number of participants in 2021 reached 32, with some states scheduled to join at a later date. The licensing standards among participating states are aligned so that any nurse in good standing in participating states can apply for the multistate license, allowing nurses to provide telehealth, travel nursing, and disaster relief in multiple states.

94. D: The most vulnerable time period for nurses is 6-12 months after joining the workforce because stress levels tend to increase, so programs that are shorter miss the time period when the program is most needed. These programs typically include clinical immersion with a strong preceptorship and scheduled learning activities.

95. B: A key principle of telehealth triage is to consider every call life-threatening regardless of how trivial it may seem initially. Remember that patients may not always address their primary concern in the beginning or may be unaware of important information that should be shared, so thorough questioning is essential. Although decision support tools are helpful, they should not be depended on instead of personal judgment. The ambulatory care nurse should never accept individual self-diagnosis, but should also not completely dismiss it, because patients are sometimes right. Frequent contacts may be necessary in some circumstances.

96. C: When creating a series of educational posters for patients utilizing three different colors, the primary color (usually the background color) should comprise about 70% of the display. Colors should not be used in the same proportions; and, if a third color is utilized, it should be used only for highlighting. The more colors that are used, the more complicated and confusing the text may seem to patients. Pictures or simple illustrations should be used on posters whenever possible.

97. C: Team-based care involves two or more healthcare providers working collaboratively to provide care to patients, families, or communities with the patient at the center of the collaboration. Teams are usually composed of multidisciplinary professionals, including nurses, physicians, therapists (physical, recreational, occupational, or rehabilitation), and social workers. A shared electronic health record is an important part of team-based care.

98. D: The vaccine is given in two doses, with the second dose given 2-6 months after the first dose. Shingrix provides greater than 90% effectiveness against shingles and postherpetic neuralgia, and it remains almost as effective for persons older than age 70. Some people experience mild flu-like symptoms after the vaccination.

99. B: Following cataract surgery, weight lifting is generally prohibited for 4-6 weeks because blood pressure increases during weight lifting and this can affect the eye. Typically, patients are advised to avoid bending over or lifting anything weighing greater than 5-10 pounds. Additionally, swimming is prohibited because patients should avoid getting any water in the operative eye (including while showering). They must also avoid rubbing the eye and avoid dust, which may cause irritation.

100. D: The primary purpose of harm-reduction principles in nursing is to decrease the negative effects of unhealthy behaviors. For example, a needle exchange program aims to decrease transmission of disease rather than to decrease addiction. Harm-reduction principles are most often applied with substance abuse, although they may be applicable to other areas as well; for example, safe-sex programs that provide condoms and sex education differ from programs that stress abstinence only. Programs based on harm-reduction principles often face opposition from those who believe that there are moral or legal issues involved.

101. A: If a patient was stung by a bee and the stinger remains in the skin, the best way to remove the stinger is to scrape a sharp instrument over the skin or wipe the area with a 4×4-inch gauze pad. It is important to remove the stinger because a granuloma may form around the stinger and may result in epidermal necrosis. Squeezing the tissue or using tweezers may result in the stinger releasing more venom.

102. B: Approximately 33% of patients who experience a TIA will have a stroke within a year, with approximately half of these having the stroke within 24 hours, so immediate treatment of a TIA is essential. TIAs are characterized by neurological symptoms (weakness, confusion, and disorientation) persisting for fewer than 24 hours. First-line treatment usually includes antiplatelet agents, such as aspirin and clopidogrel. Other treatments may include antihypertensives and, in some cases, anticoagulants, such as warfarin.

103. A: The nurse expects to constrain the uninvolved arm in order to force use of the weakened arm 90% of the day. CIMT also includes massed practice. The uninvolved arm is often restrained by placing an oven mitt on the hand. Practice is usually done for 6 hours five times a week. CIMT may be used for upper or lower extremities that retain some movement.

104. D: Trauma from running in tight shoes often causes irritation to the retrocalcaneal bursa (which is located between the Achilles tendon and the calcaneus). The tendocalcaneal bursa (which is located at the back of the heel between the calcaneus and the soft tissue) may also become inflamed.

105. D: The physician takes on the risk of liability. The nurse can be present for the consent and ensure that the consent is received in an appropriate fashion, but the ultimate responsibility for providing information to the client and attaining their consent is the physician's.

106. C: The most likely diagnosis is fat pad contusion (a.k.a. policeman's heel). Marching can compress the fat pad at the bottom of the heel, pushing it to the side of the heel and reducing the cushion. Other common causes are running on hard surfaces or up steep inclines. Treatment includes rest and shock-absorbing insoles.

107. B: The four primary principles of motivational interviewing are:

- Support of self-efficacy: Help the patient come to the realization that change is possible.
- Expression of empathy: Show appreciation and understanding for the patient's perceptions.
- Acceptance of resistance: Avoid conflict with the patient when the patient shows resistance to change.
- Examination of discrepancies: Help the patient to recognize the discrepancy between goals and behavior.

Strategies include avoiding yes/no questions, providing affirmations, providing reflective listening, summarizing, and encouraging change talk.

108. A: Although there may be many reasons why this behavior has occurred, the ambulatory care nurse should determine whether there are socioeconomic factors, such as lack of finances or transportation, that are playing a part in the patient's behavior.

109. C: The most common type of fracture in the postmenopausal woman is the vertebral fracture, outnumbering hip fractures by a ratio of 3:1. Vertebral fractures are associated with osteoporosis. Patients are often undiagnosed but complain of back pain and show spinal deformities and increased loss of height. On the other hand, wrist fractures in males are more common than vertebral fractures as an indication of osteoporosis.

110. C: ABNs are written notices issued to Fee-For-Service beneficiaries before providing items or services that Medicare won't pay for. If a Medicare patient has requested referral for acupuncture to treat chronic pain, an Advance Beneficiary Notice (ABN) may be voluntarily issued to the patient to notify the patient of non-coverage, but the ABN is not required because acupuncture is never covered by Medicare, and ABN's apply to items or services that are usually covered by Medicare but will not be covered because they are deemed not medically necessary.

111. A: The most important factor in decreasing delays in reimbursement for insurance claims is to obtain accurate demographic information about patients, including current addresses. Demographic information should be verified at each visit because, if this information is incorrect or does not match information that the insurance company has, the claim will be denied or sent back for further information. Studies have shown that more than a third of denied claims relate to inaccurate information about the patient.

112. C: The edematous area is measured for induration (hardness and swelling), not the erythematous area. Positive findings are as follows:

Induration	Interpretation
≥5 mm	Positive for immunocompromised individuals (post transplant, HIV positive) or those taking immunosuppressants.
≥10 mm	Positive for recent (<5 years) immigrants from countries with a high prevalence of tuberculosis, injection drug users, those with high-risk clinical conditions, residents/employees in high-risk environments, and mycobacteriology lab staff. Also positive for children exposed to adults who are at high risk.
>15 mm	Always a positive finding.

113. C: Intimate partner abuse does not generally require mandatory reporting; however, in most states, if injuries are caused by gunshot or knife wounds, these must be reported, so there is some overlap with intimate partner abuse. Suspected child abuse, elder abuse, and vulnerable adult abuse must always be reported. Some states require that victims of intimate partner abuse be provided referrals to resources, such as safe houses. Vulnerable adult abuse includes patients who are mentally or physically disabled.

114. D: The most critical intervention for a patient with high-altitude cerebral edema or other high-altitude sicknesses is descent to a lower elevation. The necessary descent is at least 2,000 feet (610 meters). A portable hyperbaric chamber can be used if immediate descent is not possible, but it is important to avoid any delays. Oxygen should be administered to maintain the oxygen saturation level to more than 90%. Acetazolamide may be effective for mild symptoms of acute mountain sickness. Dexamethasone is used for moderate to severe acute mountain sickness and for high-altitude cerebral edema, but it is a less critical intervention than descent to a lower elevation.

115. C: These individuals are usually paid a fixed amount. *Locum tenens* most often refers to physicians, but the term may also apply to nursing staff. *Locum tenens* medical staffers are especially important with the current shortage of physicians and nurses and for rural areas that have difficulty attracting permanent workers. Although hourly pay tends to be higher than with other types of arrangements, *locum tenens* workers often provide a financial advantage because the medical provider is able to serve patients without interruption.

116. A: Primary polycythemia is characterized by increased red blood cells with the cause being unknown. It is commonly treated with hydroxyurea, which slows production of red blood cells in the bone marrow. Interferon is also sometimes used to decrease the red blood cell count. In addition, periodic phlebotomies may be carried out to lower the concentration of red blood cells in the bloodstream. Patients must be encouraged to maintain good hydration.

117. C: If the hemoglobin and the red cell count are within normal limits, then the hematocrit is usually about three times the hemoglobin: $14 \times 3 = 42$.

Age/gender	Hemoglobin (g/dL)	Hematocrit (%)
Newborns	14.5–24.5	44–64
Children (1–6)	9.5–14.1	30–40
Adult males	14.0–17.5	45–52
Adult females	12.0–16.0	36–48

118. B: These values suggest that the patient has a bacterial infection. The WBC (>10,000), the bands (>10%), and the neutrophils are all elevated, and the lymphocyte count is decreased, which are typical signs of bacterial infection. Normal values are as follows:

Age	WBC ($\times 10^3$)	Bands %	Neut/segs %	Eos %	Baso %	Lymph %	Mono %
Newborn	9.0–30.0	10–18	36–62	0–2	0–1	26–36	0–6
1–6 yrs	5.0–19.0	5–11	13–33	0–3	0–0	46–76	0–5
Adults	5.0–10.0	3–6	50–62	0–3	0–1	25–40	3–7

119. D: With computerized learning, student attention is often focused on technology, so this strategy allows for one-on-one instruction with individual learners as the instructor sees the need or the learner requests, and the instructor is more able to monitor individual progress. However, a disadvantage is that many learners may have the same questions, so the instructor may waste time answering the same questions multiple times to individual students.

120. B: The blood sample must be placed on the test strip within 15 seconds of obtaining the sample. Therefore, it is important to ensure that the test strips are checked and the equipment is ready before obtaining the blood sample. When the patient's finger (the most common site) is used to obtain a blood sample, the patient must wash the hands thoroughly before the puncture, and the ambulatory care nurse should massage the fingertip to encourage blood flow before lancing.

121. A: Episodic care, the hallmark of ambulatory care, is characterized by being one-time or limited care so that an ongoing professional relationship is not expected. Typical examples of episodic care include visits to urgent care and outpatient surgery in an ambulatory care center. Episodic care tends to be of high volume and more unpredictable than other types of care but with more patient and family involvement. Episodic care often requires highly specialized teams of healthcare providers.

122. C: Violent and aggressive behavior is most likely to occur with long-term abuse of crack cocaine, which is more addictive than regular cocaine and produces a high that is short lasting, so the user is often constantly trying to get another hit. Most crack cocaine users begin by using cocaine, but crack cocaine tends to be less costly in the beginning; however, the increasing need for more and more frequent hits can raise the cost rapidly. Crack cocaine is cocaine that is mixed with ammonia or baking soda and heated to a solid form ("rock") that can be smoked or melted and injected.

123. D: Bloom ranked six elements from lowest complexity to highest:

- Knowledge (lowest complexity): Recalling information.
- Comprehension: Understanding information.
- Application: Using information.
- Analysis: Identifying patterns and trends.
- Synthesis: Building on old information to create new ideas.
- Evaluation (highest complexity): Assessing and judging, making recommendations.

124. A: The ambulatory care nurse should immediately report concerns to a supervisor but should not accuse the coworker directly. There may be behavioral signs (e.g., taking frequent bathroom breaks, coming to work early and staying late, and volunteering to work overtime) and workplace signs (patients' pain is unrelieved, there are broken vials, and drug choices or dosages are inappropriate for the patients).

125. C: The primary purpose of a preanesthetic medical examination is to conduct a risk assessment in order to ensure that the surgical procedure is appropriate for the patient. The timing of the preanesthetic medical examination may vary. For example, it may be carried out when the procedure is scheduled (and this may be days or weeks in advance) or immediately prior to the procedure. A history and physical evaluation are required by the American Society of Anesthesiologists for anyone who is to receive an anesthetic.

126. B: This patient would be classified as experiencing moderate anxiety. Levels of anxiety are as follows:

- **Mild**: Sharpened senses, wide perceptual field, good problem solving but may have irritability, insomnia, hypersensitivity to noise, and nervousness ("butterflies" in the stomach).
- **Moderate**: Difficulty concentrating and focusing attention; narrow perceptual field that includes only the immediate task; and episodes of dry mouth, GI upset, diaphoresis, and palpitations.
- **Severe**: Impaired concentration and inability to solve problems or complete tasks. Behavior is aimed at resolving anxiety; may exhibit dread, horror, and ritualistic behavior; and may experience GI upset, vertigo, tachycardia, and chest pain.
- **Panic**: Perceptual field is limited to self, and perceptions are distorted; unable to think rationally. May experience delusions/hallucinations and have suicidal ideation. The primary response is fight or flight.

127. D: Procrastination is a maladaptive response to stress and anxiety. Maladaptive responses also include multitasking, inadequate time management, poor listening skills, insistence on independence, compulsive behaviors, blaming others, denial, debt, poor self-care, and substance abuse. Patients may use a variety of mental processes to deal with stress, including setting expectations (positive or negative), mental imagery, self-talk (positive or negative), perfectionism, controlling behavior, and anger.

128. D: The circulating nurse often has the most interaction with the patient and may be the first nurse that the patient sees. The circulating nurse must also serve as an advocate for the patient. The scrub nurse is responsible for preparing instruments and equipment, verifying instrument counts (along with the circulating nurse), handing instruments to the surgeon, and participating in a procedural pause.

129. B: Hand washing, hand sanitizer, and gloves are standard procedure for infection control and are universal precautions to protect the nurse and the patient. These are mandated for nursing units and are not based on personal preference. Isolation protocols (such as contact and droplet precautions) may include gowns, masks, or hand washing with soap, depending on the type of isolation being used.

130. D: The first step that the nurse should advise the patient to do is to set a quit date, then to tell family and friends, and (when the date arrives) to remove all smoking supplies from the environment. The patient should also discuss the use of smoking cessation aids (such as nicotine gum) with the physician. The patient should have a support system in place and should try to keep busy on the quit day. Sucking on candy or holding or chewing something may help with cravings. Avoiding triggers is especially important, so patients may initially need to avoid smoking environments and friends who smoke.

131. B: The four characteristics that define hazardous waste materials are:

- Ignitable: Combustible/Flammable materials because of liquid flashpoints of less than 60 °C (140 °F) or chemical reaction or friction resulting in fire.
- Corrosive: pH of less than 2 or greater than 12.5 and able to burn skin or dissolve metal.
- Reactive: Explosion resulting from chemical reaction with exposure to air, water, or other material. May generate toxic gases.
- Toxic: Heavy metal compounds.

132. C: The sign-in sheet cannot contain any information about the reason for the appointment because others signing in would be privy to this health information. Sign-in sheets are allowed to contain the following information:

- Date and arrival time
- Patient's name
- Time of the appointment
- Healthcare provider's name

#	Name	Appt time	Arrival time	Appt. with	New (√)
1	Terry Jamison	8:30	8:20	Dr. stephens	
2	M. J. Malek	9:00	8:55	Dr. Stephens	√
3	Lucy Madsen	9:00	8:45	Dr. Rubin	

133. A: With central sleep apnea, an underlying condition (such as heart failure, cardiopulmonary disease, or stroke) causes the sleep apnea, so that the central nervous system does not trigger respirations in response to changes in the level of oxygen. Cheyne-Stokes breathing is a common finding, with rapid respirations and increased oxygen saturation alternating with apneic periods and falling oxygen saturation.

134. C: If a physician in a clinic was delayed, resulting in three patients having to reschedule appointments after waiting for extended periods, the first step necessary for service recovery is to apologize. This should be done early in the waiting period rather than the end and, if the physician is delayed more than 15 minutes, another appointment should be scheduled then rather than having the patients wait longer. It's important to listen to the patient and express empathy and to offer some type of atonement, such as free parking, if possible.

135. B: This statement is probably an indication of caregiver stress, which often exhibits as anger or frustration. Other signs of caregiver stress include depression, denial, anxiety, and social withdrawal. Caregivers are often exhausted and sleep poorly, contributing to irritability, poor concentration, and health problems.

136. C: Functional status for patients with rheumatoid arthritis:

Functional status (rheumatoid arthritis)	
Class 1	Can independently carry out activities of daily living.
Class 2	Can carry out usual activities (self-care and work) but limited in other activities (sports and household chores).
Class 3	Can carry out usual activities involving self-care but limited in work and other activities.
Class 4	Limited in ability to carry out all usual activities involving self-care, work, and other activities.

137. B: Costs are generally lower, which is especially important if the person is uninsured. This is especially important if the person is uninsured. Wait times may also be shorter, although this may not be true of all urgent care centers. Hospitals usually have more up-to-date equipment and equipment, such as computed tomography and magnetic resonance imaging scanners, as well as onsite laboratory testing not typically available in urgent care centers because of cost.

138. A: If a patient with diabetes takes insulin, this type of therapy is classified as replacement because the insulin replaces the natural insulin that is deficient or absent. Prophylactic therapy, such as with perioperative antibiotics, is intended to prevent illness. Acute therapy, such as with epinephrine, is intended to treat an acute or severe illness. Palliative therapy, such as with an antiemetic, is used to provide comfort rather than curative treatment.

139. D: If a patient complains of postmastectomy breast pain syndrome, this is an example of differentiation, a type of neuropathic pain. Patients may experience pain, burning, numbness, and tingling in the breast, axilla, and arm. Differentiation also accounts for phantom pain associated with limb amputation. Other types of neuropathic pain include central (from a primary lesion, such as stroke), peripheral neuropathies (postherpetic neuralgia, trigeminal neuralgia, diabetic neuropathy), and sympathetically maintained pain, which results from activity of the sympathetic nervous system, such as with complex regional pain syndrome.

140. C: Staples for facial lacerations are usually removed earlier, in 3-5 days, and staples for the scalp in 5-7 days. For other areas of the body, 7-10 days or more is the usual. A longer duration may result in scarring and infection from retained staples. A staple removal tool is used to remove the staples.

141. A: Injury during the commute to and from work is not covered by workers' compensation insurance, but injury at a mandatory-attendance company-sponsored sports activity, during travel for company-sponsored business, and in the parking lot while walking into the building are all covered. If injury results from violation of policies, intentional or illegal acts, or horseplay, this type of injury is also not covered. Workers' compensation insurance provides three different types of benefits: cash to replace lost wages, reimbursement for medical costs associated with the injury, and death benefits to survivors.

142. B: The first step is to soak the digit in warm povidone-iodine or antiseptic soap solution for 5 minutes. Then, the digit is positioned and draped with sterile 4×4-inch gauze pads to collect blood and the cautery needle is activated. When the cautery needle is hot, it is applied at a 90-degree angle to the nail at the middle of the hematoma and is held until resistance is no longer felt and the needle has penetrated the nail. The cautery needle is removed, and the blood is allowed to drain.

143. C: If an older female patient with moderately advanced dementia is cradling a doll and says, "This is my baby," and refuses to relinquish the doll for an examination, the most appropriate response is: "I won't bother your baby." The confusion associated with dementia is different from hallucinations or delusions experienced by those with mental illness, so arguing and trying to correct or reason with the patient is usually not helpful and may lead to agitation and aggressive behavior.

144. C: The center cannot ask the patient to bring someone to assist and should examine the patient in the wheelchair only if sitting during examination is appropriate for the type of problem that the patient has. All ambulatory care centers should have wheelchair-accessible examination tables or gurneys or appropriate lifts available.

145. B: If the ambulatory care nurse has called a patient who is being treated for chronic depression because the patient has missed one appointment and two sessions of the support group, the statement by the patient that is of most concern is: "I've been giving all my things away, and I feel so much better." Patients suffering from depression who decide to commit suicide often begin to give away their things and claim that they feel better, and may even appear calmer and more relaxed, but these are warning signs.

146. D: A just culture differentiates among:

- **Human error**: Inadvertent actions, mistakes, or lapses in proper procedure. Management includes considering processes, procedures, training, or design to determine the cause of the error as well as consoling the person.
- **At-risk behavior**: Unjustified risk or choice. Management includes providing incentives for correct behavior and disincentives for incorrect behavior and coaching the person.
- **Reckless behavior**: Conscious disregard for proper procedures. Management includes remedial action and/or punitive action.

147. B: Following fine-needle aspiration of a breast lesion, patient instructions should include applying a pressure dressing and ice packs for 24 hours to prevent development of a hematoma. Patients often experience moderate pain, which is usually relieved with acetaminophen taken every 4 hours. Patients should also be advised to immediately report any indications of infection, such as swelling and redness, discharge, fever, foul odor, or increased pain after 24 hours.

148. A: In ambulatory care, the individual most in control of patient care is the patient him- or herself. Healthcare personnel's contact with patients is limited (usually less than 24 hours and often measured in minutes); therefore, most of the responsibility for following medical advice regarding treatment lies with the patient, so the patient's understanding and motivation are critical elements in recovery. Therefore, it is important to treat the patient as a collaborator throughout the process of evaluation and care.

149. B: In this situation, it is critical that adrenal crisis be suspected and immediately treated without waiting for confirming tests, because the condition is life-threatening. The first step in treatment should be to administer 100 mg of hydrocortisone IV over 30 seconds, and then 1,000 mL of 5% dextrose in 0.9% saline solution containing 100 mg of hydrocortisone over a 2-hour period, followed by treatment according to protocol.

150. B: Span of control refers to the number of individuals that a person supervises or receives reports from within an organization. A wide span of control (a large number of subordinates) is common when workers are involved in routine work, because the need for supervision is minimal. However, with very complex tasks, a narrow span of control is usually necessary. Factors to consider when determining the span of control include the size of the organization, the skills of the workers, the culture of the organization, and the training and responsibilities of the supervisors.

It's Your Moment, Let's Celebrate It!

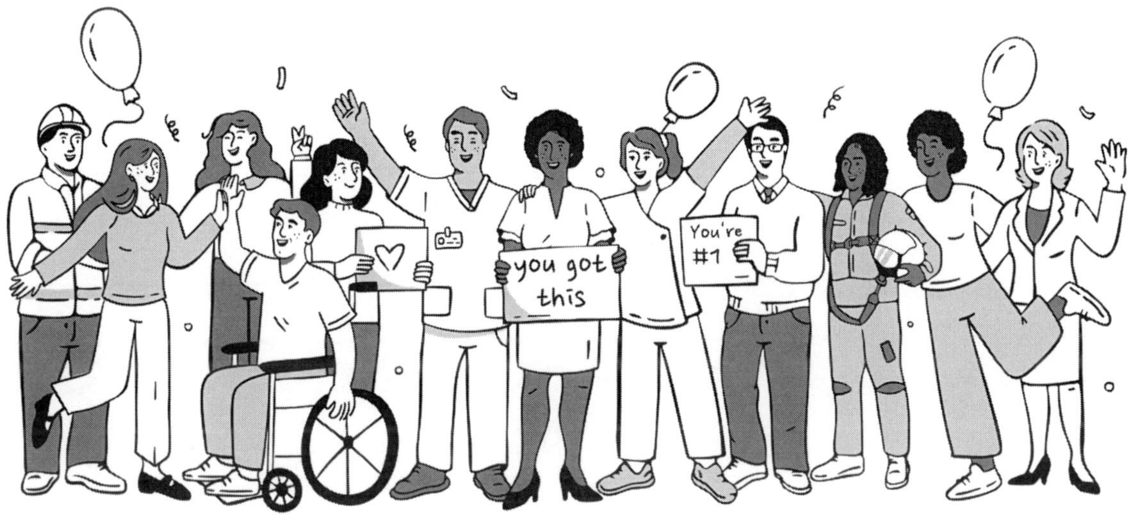

Share your story @mometrixtestpreparation